The *SHE* Book of Slimming

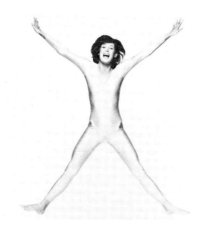

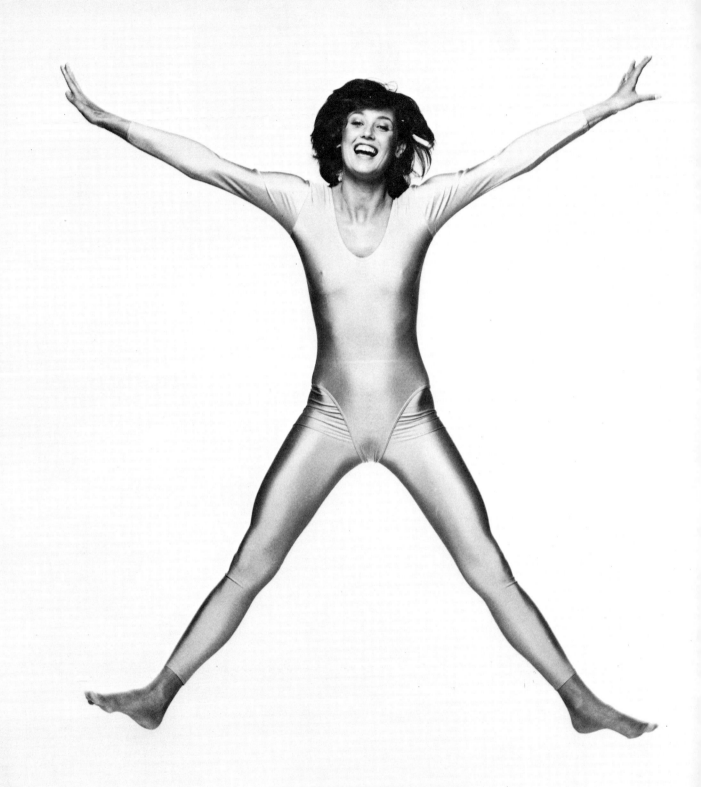

The **SHE**
Book of Slimming

Sally Ann Voak

Arthur Barker Limited / Ebury Press

London

Published in Great Britain by
Arthur Barker Ltd (A subsidiary of Weidenfeld (Publishers) Ltd)
91 Clapham High Street, London SW4 7TA
and
Ebury Press
National Magazine House, 72 Broadwick Street, London W1V 2BP

ISBN 0 213 16802 2 cased
ISBN 0 213 16807 3 paperback
Set, printed and bound in Great Britain by
Fakenham Press Limited, Fakenham, Norfolk

Contents

5 Exercising

Acknowledgements

The illustrations in this book are reproduced by courtesy of the following:

Beverly Goodway: 1, 2, 8, 12, 22, 65–8, 72, 78, 79, 83–105, 111
Lee Higham: 71
Chris Holland: 21
Transworld Features: 25, 28, 34, 62, 80
Weidenfeld and Nicolson Archive: 14 (Joy FitzSimmons), 15–17 (Rosalyn Toohig), 19 and 31 (Marcia Fenwick), 38–56 (Elizabeth Watkins)

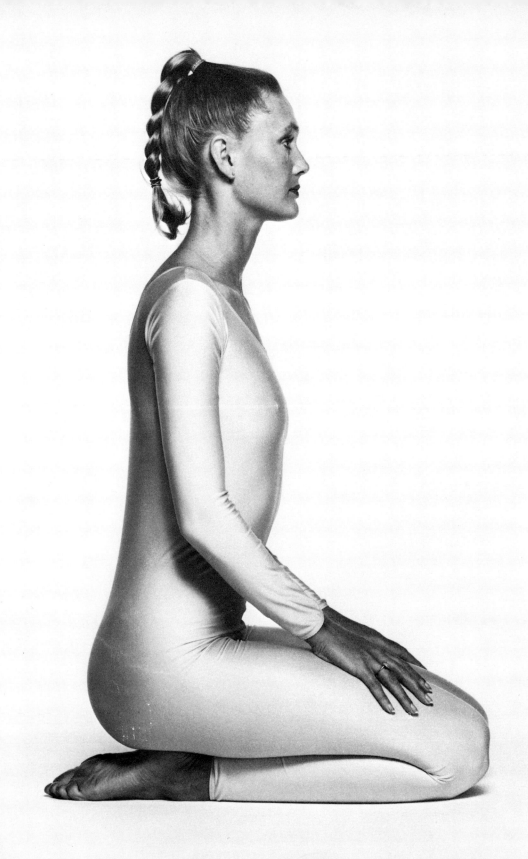

Introduction

This book is all about bodies; shape, health, performance and that smashing word *vitality*, which seems to combine energy, attractiveness, joie de vivre, good looks, happiness. It's about *your* body in particular; whether it's youngish, older, slim, middling or frankly fat. The *SHE* philosophy is that a body should first and foremost be *healthy*; in the magazine, we don't keep nagging about slimming until we're all sick to death of counting calories. Instead, we aim to provide guidelines for enjoyable living, exercising, even eating, which are geared to help you make the very best of your body.

Nowadays, you don't have to be thin to be beautiful. In fact the very best-looking, most glamorous people are often very curvy indeed. If you're a large-framed, tall person with size 12 shoes (male or female!), then there is no way that you are going to look *thin*; the only way you're likely to look if you over-diet is *ill*. Similarly, if you're tiny with bird-like bones and teeny feet, it simply won't do to carry an elephant's share of flesh. What you should aim for is a body shape and size that's aesthetically pleasing, with good proportions and firm muscular tone. Almost anyone (except those with psychological and/or physiological problems which inhibit weight control) can achieve this by following a nutritious, non-boring diet and taking some kind of regular exercise. The psychological motivation for achieving maximum body shape potential is important too; you've got to *want* to be attractive, and to love yourself enough to enjoy paying yourself the attention you deserve!

In this book I'll be explaining all about the latest diets and exercise routines, but the ultimate 'expert' will be *you*. For you, after all, know your body best of all!

Your shape 'Shape' is one of those overworked words in the world of keeping fit and healthy. But when you consider what it *really* means (the total effect produced by an object or person's outline), you start to realize just how much the 'ideal' shape has altered in the last hundred years or so. For women, it's progressed from the ample bosom and tiny waistline of the Victorians through the flat-chested look of the twenties and the willowy figure of the thirties to the stockyness of the war years and the almost emaciated thinness of the sixties. At last, in the eighties, the shape of an 'ideal' woman has become curvier, more rounded and healthier-looking. For men, the portly tummy and watch-chain-festooned waistcoat of the Victorian and Edwardian gentleman switched to a more dapper, much slimmer look during the twenties and thirties; wartime fellas seemed ample-bottomed (those baggy trousers perhaps), broad-

Exercise helps you beat *stress* as well as tone up your muscles.

shouldered, and shorter than the post-war trendies of the fifties and early sixties. The fashion for tight jeans in the late sixties and seventies seemed to breed a whole race of young men with tiny bottoms, skinny legs, and high voices! Happily, they've filled out a little these days – although perhaps things have gone a bit too far; I notice more and more fat tummies on *younger* men (lager advertising has a lot to answer for!) and a general thickening-up of the male shape.

If you can stand the shock, check out your own shape by standing, naked, in front of a large, full-length mirror (this is an exercise which should carry a government health warning!) with the light *behind* you. You will then see a sharp outline of the shape you present to your loved ones in your most intimate moments. I'll say no more at this stage. . . .

Your health and your weight You only need to be about ten per cent over the top of the 'ideal' weight for your height and frame to start running a serious risk of undermining your health. High blood pressure, heart disease, diabetes, back trouble, respiratory infections – they all tend to gang up on the overweight. So what's 'ideal'? Charts produced by life insurance companies are based on life-expectancy statistics, so they do give a reasonable guide to the correct weight for *you*. However, the mirror test I've just mentioned probably gives a far more realistic view of the state of your figure than the scales in your bathroom. If you've put on weight over the last few years then you know, in your heart of hearts, that you could, and should, weigh less. You may have noticed that as the pounds pile on so have the nagging little health problems like breathlessness, aches and creaks, heart palpitations, lethargy, accident-proneness. Sorry, things can only get *worse*. For, as we get older, our calorie needs are less and our taste for good food stays the same – hence creeping fat! If, by the time you reach your forties or fifties, you are 20 per cent overweight, or more, then you could really be in trouble healthwise. Okay, we all know about the happy, energetic fatties who enjoy life . . . but, apart from Cyril Smith and Sophie Tucker, there aren't *that* many of them around, are there? Unless you plan to spend your retirement queueing up for a prescription at the doctor's surgery and watching television, it makes sense to trim back those dangerous extra inches before it becomes much more difficult to do so. Personally, I intend to spend my sixties and seventies travelling the world (piloting my own plane, of course) and I really won't have *time* for health problems. Being slim, therefore, makes sound sense.

What performance means to you I often wonder what some of the more frenzied jogging fans plan to *do* once they reach a really high level of fitness and endurance. Will they become marathon runners, mountaineers, swim the Atlantic? Obviously, if you're an Olympic athlete the level of performance which you demand from your body will be very great indeed – far greater than that needed by your average sedentary worker. I maintain that fitness should be attained to the level that's right for your life, and for most of us that's a fairly modest level. A regular exercise routine, some enjoyable sports, and a fair amount of walking (or gentle jogging, if you *must* show off) are all you need to be able to cope with the maximum strains which life may demand from you: the exertions of gardening, running for the bus, summer swimming, dancing.

It's important to *enjoy* keeping fit, and it's also a good idea to choose exercises and sports that help tone up muscles which may become neglected because of your work. If you're a writer or other bum-bashing sedentary worker like me, than your buttock muscles are obviously a sitting target (sorry!) for the dreaded spreads. Walking, swimming, skating, football or squash all help to get our bums in shape. If you're a shop worker, clippie, factory worker or other 'standing-up' type, then a spot of horse-riding, rock-climbing or archery would help to give your arms and waistline a whirl, and some tennis or golf would help loosen up any backstrain caused by all that standing around!

Also to be considered is the 'high' that exercise gives you. When your lungs have to work harder, there is a definite boost of oxygen to the *brain*, which works wonders for jaded minds. A group of journalists I know who go to a regular lunchtime dance class are so bright in the afternoons that they make the others in their office feel positively dim by comparison! They glow with energy and radiate original thoughts . . . they are also slim and attractive.

How do you decide your own performance 'ideal'? Test yourself: aim to swim five lengths or run half a mile, neither of which should be difficult for you. Stop when you feel tired. Didn't make it? You *definitely* need to boost your energy levels.

Vitality It's vital if you want to enjoy life! How many times have you refused an invitation, put off a job, been gloomy, doomy or despondent? Too many? You need an injection of *vitality* into your life. The dictionary defines it as 'persistent energy' . . . and when it says persistent, it could mean that it's the kind of energy which manages to remain buoyant despite the state of the economy, the awful weather, the latest train strike, or the combined challenges of pre-menstrual tension, hassles at work and a reminder from Barclaycard. Honest, if you can bounce back smiling from that lot, than you have *vitality*! Seriously, I would hate to miss out on any of life's pleasures – from sex to playing soccer in the park – because I felt too bored or dreary to enjoy them. Vitality is about optimism, having fun, feeling good – it's also about eating well, taking regular exercise and making the most of your *body*. It's the opposite of boredom – and so is this book!

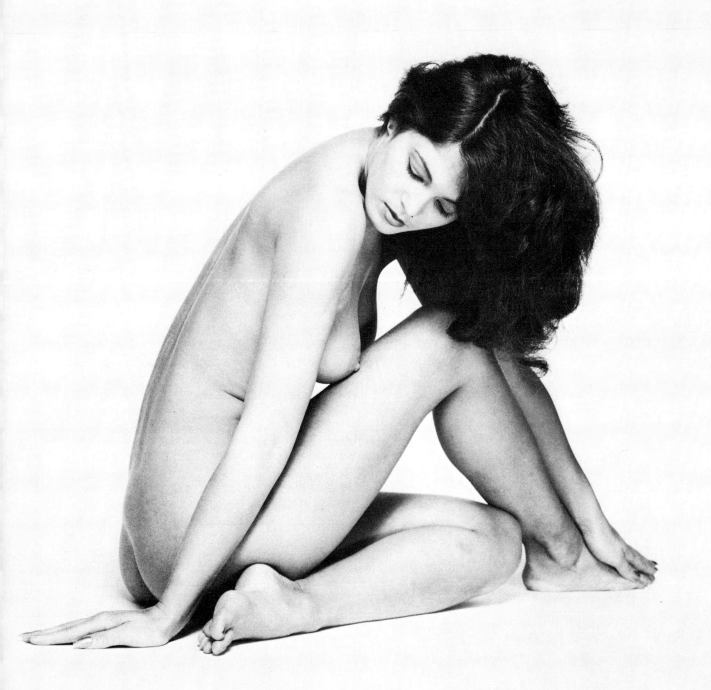

1 Body Assessment

You can blame your *parents* for at least some of the things you hate about your body, but you should blame *yourself* for the vast majority of them! The basic shape and bone-structure you've inherited will, of course, determine the framework of your figure; the things you can alter are the amount of flesh covering that framework, the tone and strength of your muscles, and the mobility of your limbs and joints. The latter is perhaps the most important of all: creaky joints when you're young become even creakier as you get older. It's no fun to be bedridden or disabled by back trouble; it's been estimated that 300 *million* working days are lost through this problem each year.

Your figure

You are likely to fall into one of three general categories (these are only a guide – everyone's different): the ectomorph (lanky, slender and usually slim); the mesomorph (strong, muscular, with large bone and muscle development) and endomorph (soft, rounded tum, small chest, hands and feet). Both the latter categories are prone to being overweight, and the poor old endomorph most likely of all.

Check out your type by standing naked in front of a long mirror. If you're tall, with delicate bone structure under those fatty layers, then you're the ectomorph type and should aim to be slim, erect and graceful (Gayle Hunnicutt is a typical ectomorph, and you'll be delighted to know that she has to diet constantly to remain sylphlike). If your shoulders are broad, your midriff fairly flat and your hips wide, plus a good, full bosom, then you're the mesomorph type. You may well feel that this is a desperately unjust state of affairs – you look *huge*, even when only slightly overweight. You should aim to be firm-muscled and compact rather than slim, and you should develop super posture and controlled movements to avoid the 'fairy elephant' nickname you probably had to endure through childhood. (Margaux Hemingway is a mesomorph; she'll never weigh eight stone, but through sensible dieting and exercise – which is popular with mesomorphs – she looks wonderful. So can *you*.) It's probably a mistake for the chunky mesomorph to use the scales too often, for ten stone may sound depressingly fat compared with the eight stone targets of your endomorph chums. You should, however, check for flesh firmness and muscle tone by observing your shape constantly and by doing the 'finger and thumb test': grabbing folds of spare flesh at strategic places – tummy, tops of thighs, hips, upper arms – and making sure that the amount you can pinch is a one-inch chunk or less.

Every body is, potentially, a graceful, beautiful one.

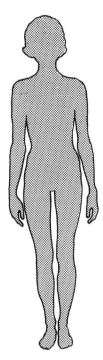
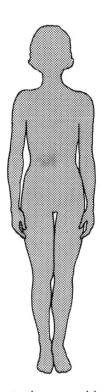
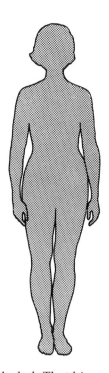

From left, basic shapes of ectomorph, mesomorph and endomorph.

And so to the poor old endomorph, me included. That hippy look and those smallish breasts are definitely not enhanced by the soft, round, sticking-out tummy we so often have to live with. Actually, we *don't*. The secret of making the most of this figure-type is to minimize hips and tummy with exercise and diet, and maximize breasts with perking-up exercises (see page 102). According to psychologist W. H. Sheldon, who first coined the three body types, the endomorph's character centres around food and comfort. Right! Ask our noblest endomorph, HM the Queen – luckily she is surrounded by such a surfeit of *both* that she's able to place her mind on higher things. That's why her figure has remained reasonably trim throughout a life of ten-course banquets, soft sofas and after-dinner mints.

So much for the body type you inherit; what happens to it next? Don't think about your fiendish food intake yet, that just piles on extra flesh. No, right now we're concerned with three big influences on your shape: gravity, environment, movement.

Forces to fight against

Gravity Ever thought of your daily life as a constant battle against the force of gravity? It acts upon us at every moment of our existence; sitting, standing, during all movement, even when we're lying down in bed asleep. If you stand or sit badly your body has to work extra hard to

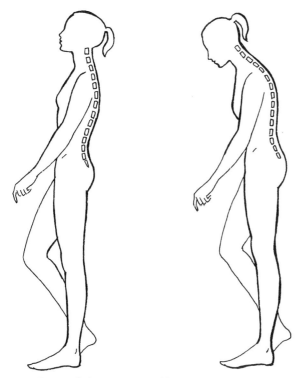

remain upright, and the irrepressible pressure of gravity begins to distort your body, and pull it out of shape. A simple example is the woman whose rounded shoulders and pendulous breasts proclaim a constant struggle against gravity (and against the world itself).

The natural centre of gravity is a point just inside the upper part of the pelvis (the second sacral vertebra). The line of gravity is a vertical line passing through points just behind the ear, behind the shoulder joint, through the sacrum and the knee joint to a point just in front of the ankle. If you stand so this line is vertical, your posture will be correct.

Now place your feet slightly apart, and try to make your nose, chin, breastbone, navel and the front of your pelvis into an imaginary straight line which falls between your feet. Now bend your knees slightly; stretch upwards as if your head were being suspended on a string from the ceiling, and let your arms drop gently downwards, middle fingers at the outside of your thighs (pull your shoulder blades slightly backwards, if necessary). Comfy? Now just check your reflection in a long mirror. Do you notice how much slimmer you look? Your tummy is being held in, your bosom is higher, your bottom neater-looking? Practise this posture several times a day, walking around the house with arms swinging loosely forwards and backwards. Try, too, to adopt this posture when you're out for a walk (avoid throwing things out of balance by carrying a huge bag or wearing high heels). You'll be harmonizing with gravity

Correct posture (far left) and the more usual slouch. Do make a real effort to walk tall.

instead of fighting it, and the benefits will be immediate and dramatic. For instance, you may quickly notice muscular tightness (even a few aches) at the top of the thighs, on your tummy and bottom, but you'll look graceful and suffer less undue exertion. People may even remark that your diet seems to be working at last!

Environment Almost everything around you conspires to ruin your figure, from the squashy office chair you sit on at work to the low-roofed sports car your poor frame gets crunched into every day. Worst of the lot is the shopping bag: the fashion for huge hold-all type bags may be practical but it's rapidly producing a nation of hunch-shouldered, sideways-dipping people with one arm longer than the other! Is your work, home or car conspiring to ruin your figure? Check out these points:

Desks and tables Make sure they're at a comfortable height; when you're sitting on a chair, back straight, feet flat on the floor, your *bent* elbows should just touch the table top. Awful consequences of too-low desks include bulging tummies (the flesh is pressed concertina-fashion while your spine is curved), hunched shoulders, backache, neck stiffness.

Chairs Perhaps the worst figure-spoiler of all, the office chair is usually a darn sight more cruel to your body than that extra helping of jam roly-poly. If it's too high or too low, you can probably count the cricks in your neck or the rolls of fat around your waistline. If the seat is squashy (or you use a soft cushion – shame!) your bottom is probably the same. If the back is badly designed, you've probably got a nasty sinking feeling in the base

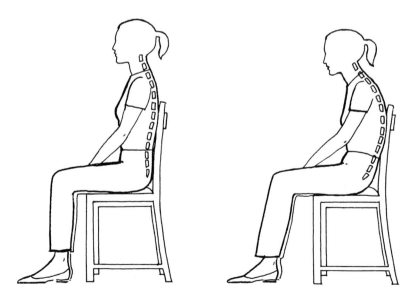

The harder the chair the easier it is to sit straight. If you must slump (far right) slump backwards, never forwards.

of your spine. So *change the chair*. The perfect model should have height requirements as described in *Desks and tables*, and a high, straightish back, firm seat and legs. Swivel chairs may have the advantage of height adjustment, but they encourage sloppy sitting and sideways leg-crossing. Ideally, you should sit with your bottom well back (try it – feel the relief in your back), your feet on the floor with the angle between thighs and calves at 90°. *Don't* twiddle your legs, cross your ankles or wrap your feet around each other. If you're watching television, beware of the big slump. The type of chair above is best for comfort, but an armchair will do if you can sit upright in it. If you like, sit on the floor, with your back against the front of an arm-chair and a small cushion behind your bottom.

Working surfaces These should be at wrist-height when you stand close to them, one foot forward, shoulders relaxed. Obviously, you can't rip out your kitchen or get your boss to re-design his shop counters if they are too high or too low. But you *can* stand on a board, footstool or plank to raise your body, or sit on a stool, chair or bench to lower it. If you're in a job which entails long hours of working at a production line or bench, these tips are really important: hunched shoulders, for instance, can lead to horrors like migraine, sciatica and headaches (bad for productivity!) as well as a rotten figure.

Cars When you're trying out a car for comfort, make sure you'll be able to drive with your knees comfortably bent, your shoulders back, and your hands and arms relaxed. You must be able to see over the wheel properly

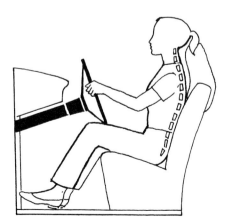
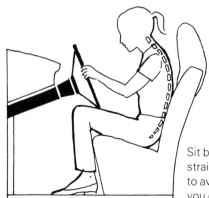

Sit back for safety and comfort – and a straight back (far left). Adjust the seat to avoid hunching your shoulders when you drive.

(sounds obvious, but you must have seen all those bods peering over the driving wheel in their cars – I know I have) and your back must be supported. Oddly enough, it's more likely to be the old-fashioned bench seat that supports your back best than the latest bucket seat. The latter can be excruciatingly uncomfortable, although bad design can be remedied slightly with a small cushion placed behind your bottom. You really should be able to sit well back in the seat *and* drive properly.

Beds It sounds masochistic but a firm bed really *does* help your figure. Soft, downy, sink-in-and-smother beds are bad for you because they simply don't give your body enough support. Gravity rears its ugly head again and, while your left leg is sinking into the mattress, your *other* muscles are working overtime to support the rest of your body. You're also likely to cuddle into a nestlike dip in a soft bed – firm mattresses are great for spreading out! If you can train yourself away from mounds of pillows, your upper body will benefit: your chin will stay single (even if you don't) and your neck will be less likely to feel cricked. Your shoulders will resist hunching, and your bosom will heave and fall gently without becoming 'pigeoned'.

Equipment You can always recognize a dentist by her legs: one's usually shorter and fatter than the other because she spends her working life bending to one side with the weight of her body pressed heavily on one leg. Oh yes, she's usually got hunched shoulders and a squint, too. Sounds horrendous? It happens. If you, like the unfortunate dentist, must work with equipment which makes you contort your body into strange shapes, you will certainly become somewhat 'deformed' *unless* you consciously try to remedy the situation with 'anti-body twisting exercises' (such as yoga asanas – see page 82) every day, and/or try to make the things you have to work with fit in with your body for a change. For instance, if the file you need constantly is located in a drawer which can only be reached if you stand on one leg, twist your body to one side and hunch your shoulders, there's a good case for moving it! Or, if your spade, shovel or hoe is too short and you have to bend over all day, there's an excellent reason for switching to a longer model. The tools of your trade can be anything from your mirror (Well lit? Well positioned?) to your child's pushchair (is it the right height?) or your computer or type-writer keyboard; check out the machine which dominates your life – it could be ruining your figure!

Movement When you say someone is a 'beautiful mover', that really *is* a compliment! We all have to move about (some, sadly, seem to move as little as possible) and the way we do so has a profound and lasting effect on our shape. Posture is important when you walk or run; aim for that 'head held high' feeling, and let your arms swing naturally and easily.

Feet are very important: strip off your shoes, socks or tights and watch yourself walk – if you tend to walk over on the insides of your feet, then fat will accumulate on the outside of your hips and thighs – it's nature's way of restoring balance. Similarly, if you walk on the outside of your feet, you'll notice fatty pads on the insides of your thighs. It's relatively simple to correct these faults: for a start, wear the right shoes with plenty of width for your toes, and support for your instep and heels, *don't* load yourself up with bags and parcels if you can help it, and choose clothes which allow freedom of movement and grace (pleated skirts, loose trousers). It's well worth investing in leather shoes which fit properly, don't cramp your toes and make walking a pleasure.

One of the best reasons for losing weight is that it makes *movement* so much more pleasurable; you can enjoy the sensation of dashing up and down stairs, running through the park, walking in the rain, all without carrying around the extra burden of weight (even half a stone extra is the equivalent to a fairly heavy shopping bag – think about it!). Luckily, movement and healthy eating go hand in hand: as you begin to adjust your eating pattern to a sensible level and the pounds begin to drop off, then you feel more like moving about. As your daily mobility level increases, your calorie-burning ability increases and it becomes easier and easier to lose weight. Don't be a lump – *move.*

Even when you're pregnant, it's important to keep moving. A pregnant woman should never stand around; even if she's at a party, she should be walking on the spot every now and then. The secret of good posture and easy movement during pregnancy is in balance adjustment to compensate for the bump in front and the spinal curve behind. In late pregnancy there's a very exaggerated sacro-lumbar curve in the lower spine; if you try to cope with it by hollowing your back still further and sticking your stomach out you'll simply waddle like a duck, and get back and shoulder aches. You should tuck in your bottom, lifting the baby into the 'cradle' of your pelvis, and tuck your buttocks together like two tight little buns. You should walk tall and swing your shoulders and arms. If you follow this walking method, you'll feel good and look several months' slimmer too. It will also be easier to get your figure back after the birth if you've been a beautiful mover beforehand. Childbirth expert Sheila Kitzinger believes in keeping on the move during labour. She says:

'Thirty or forty years ago all midwives got their patients to walk during the first stage of labour, to produce pressure from the baby's head against the cervix and use the forces of gravity to initiate birth. Nowadays hospitals tend to keep mums in labour in bed. Honestly, it's more comfortable to keep on the move; it's easier to tolerate quite powerful contractions when you're on the move, and labour is shorter.'

Movement for non-pregnant people includes such pursuits as jogging, swimming, skating, tennis, squash and badminton. To my mind, the sport that can do most for your figure is *swimming*. Although it burns off

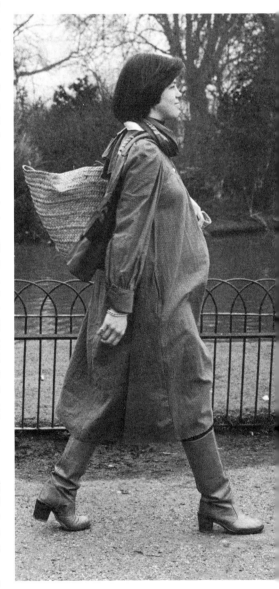

Even when pregnant, walk rather than sit in a traffic jam!

fewer calories per minute than squash or badminton, it does exercise all the main body muscles and helps develop graceful movement and posture. For a rapid and noticeable figure improvement without dieting, try swimming once or twice a week; do twelve to fifteen lengths of gentle breast-stroke, without frantic rushing, and within a month your shape will change visibly; benefits will include a prettier bustline and flatter tummy. No time? Most towns have a pool, *use* it! The routine described above takes no longer than fifteen to thirty minutes which can easily be fitted into a lunchtime or even before work.

I am not a mad-keen jogging advocate simply because I have seen so many hunched shoulders, furrowed brows and droopy bosoms on joggers frantically battling against the elements and looking less and less beautiful by the minute! If you *do* jog, wear a good supporting bra to prevent bosom-droop and develop a graceful style with head held high, shoulders back, tummy and bottom in and arms swinging naturally. Wear the right kind of shoes and socks (supportive running shoes, not old sneakers), and beware of the jogger's knee syndrome caused by the jarring effect of jogging downhill; doctors are now reporting more cases of joint damage than heart attacks! Jogging won't do much for you (in fact it could do harm) if you bounce round the block after a hectic day and heavy lunch, once a week. You need to jog regularly, three or four times a week, to feel the benefits.

Just look at yourself

Here are three tests which should give you a more honest answer to the question of your weight than your scales. Don't forget that while exercising and the firming of flabby muscles will improve your general outline, weight loss may not be dramatic. As muscle weighs more than fat some of those extra pounds won't be lost, simply redistributed.

The mirror test Stand in bra and pants – or naked if you dare! – in front of a full-length mirror, shoulders back and relaxed, hands by your sides. Now turn sideways on and study your body profile. Bulging tummy? If it sticks out even when you hold it in, you need exercise or diet and probably both. Flabby thighs? Jodhpur-shaped thighs respond well to a mixture of diet, exercise and massage. Thick upper arms? Exercise will help to tone up muscles and reduce flab. Droopy bosom and bottom? Try the exercises on pages 102–5, and check your posture against the diagram on page 15.

The skin-fold test Doctors use skin-fold testing calipers on certain parts of the body to determine excess weight. The total value of their findings is then related to body fat percentage. Ideally, an adult male should have about 15 per cent of his body in the form of fat, and a female about 25 per cent – the extra forms curves and protects the child-bearing regions!

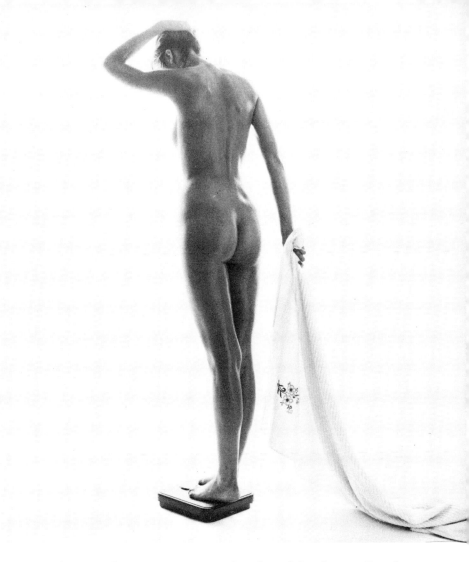

Eyes down for – a shock? The scales may depress you, but it's how you *look* and *feel* that really matters.

You can do a similar test using your thumb and forefinger. Simply pinch the maximum amount of flesh possible at these points: central midriff, tummy-button, one side of your waist-line, upper back below shoulder-blade, inside upper arm between elbow and armpit, just above hip-bone, half-way up inside thighs and fleshiest part of calves. If you can take up more than one inch of flesh at any of these points then you need to lose weight and tone up your muscles.

The swimsuit test The old idea of trying on last year's swimsuit to see if you've expanded since you bought it is still a valid way of checking your expansion. Do it a couple of months after your holiday, then again a month before the next one. If the swimsuit is frankly tight then you must take your body in hand rapidly. Don't allow the pounds to pile on gradually over the years, or it will be much harder to lose weight.

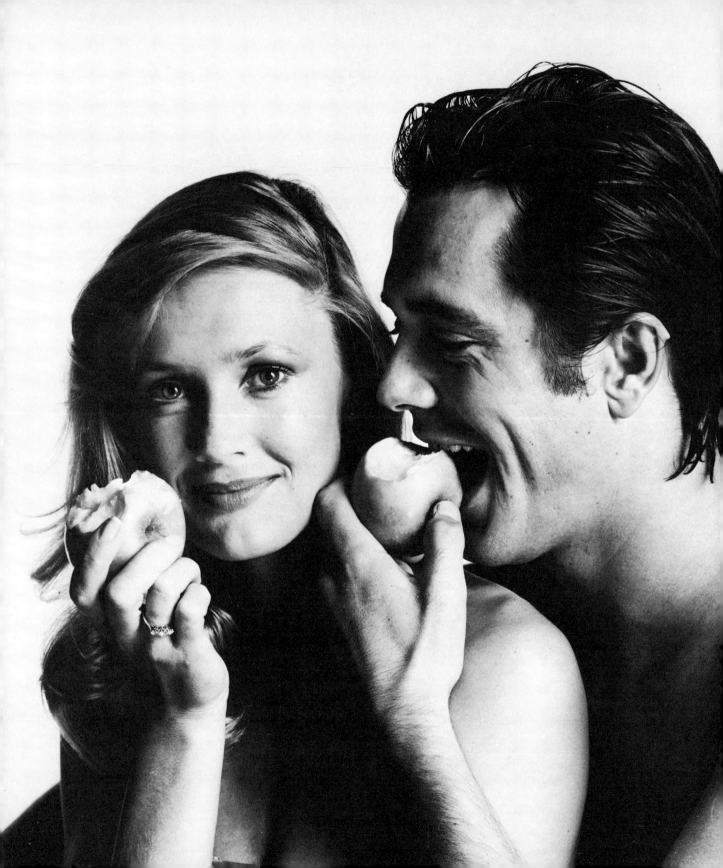

2 Eating Right

Before thinking about eating to be *slim*, think about eating to be *fit*. Are you sure you are getting your fair share of the nutrients which will keep you healthy, happy and in tip-top form all day long, every day? Although few people may actually become sick through nutritional deficiency in our society, there are many who suffer from a kind of 'sub-clinical' food deficiency which prevents them getting the most out of life. Symptoms of this are frequently poor skin, dull hair, listlessness, constant tiredness, irritability and overweight.

Food provides us with many different nutrients, and frequently these are dependent on one another to work properly in the body. That's why it makes sense to follow a diet which includes a variety of different foods, taken from the different food groups. It is not sensible to follow a strict diet which cuts out carbohydrate, for example, for any length of time since this can cause an imbalance which could potentially be dangerous. It is equally daft to deprive yourself of the chance of consuming the nutrients you need by sloppy eating: the lunchtime hamburger and chips, for instance, or the bedsitter soup and toast regime.

The major nutrients

Proteins are in meat, fish, cheese, eggs, milk, cereals and nuts. They are the essential constituents of the millions of microscopic cells which make up blood, tissue and organs. They are essential for body growth and repair. Proteins come in many different types, made up of smaller units called amino-acids. Different food proteins are complementary, so it's sensible to include a variety of different protein sources in your diet, both animal and vegetable. A healthy adult woman needs about 5g of protein daily (equivalent to about 10g of cod, or 8g lean meat, or 8g hard cheese). There are about 22 calories in every 5g of protein.

For slimmers, proteins can be valuable since they have the advantage of giving sustained energy over a long period of time. However, they are fairly high in calories; if you eat too much meat you won't lose weight!

Carbohydrates are in sugar, starchy foods, confectionery, puds, pastries, bread, cereals. The simpler carbohydrates, monosaccharides, are the sugars. Monosaccharide molecules linked together form polysaccharides, or starch, which is a more complex form of carbohydrate. They are split up, then converted into glucose which is circulated to all parts of the body via the bloodstream. Carbohydrates provide energy and calories. Unfortunately, we often consume too many carbohydrates (it's been estimated

When it comes to the crunch, an apple is better for both of you than a cream cake or bag of sweets.

that the Western diet contains about forty or fifty per cent), especially in cakes, puds and confectionery; these foods are low in other nutrients, so they should be limited on a slimming diet. Bread, potatoes and pasta, however, do contain vitamins, minerals and proteins and should be eaten in small amounts even if you are slimming.

Fats are found in foods like meat, ice-cream, and mayonnaise as well as in the main sources – butter, margarine, milk, cheese and vegetable oils. They occur in several forms: triglicyrides which are made up of chemicals called fatty acids joined on to glycerol; phospholipids such as lecithin; and sterols such as cholesterol. Their function is to provide a source of energy, make food more palatable and help you feel satisfied. They are high in calories (butter, which is mostly fat, provides 800 calories per 100g!), and current medical opinion advises that we should cut down on all forms of fat. At present, our diet is about 40–50 per cent fat – 30 per cent would be healthier. A real effort at cutting down fat levels has already been introduced in America, where significant success has been reported in controlling fat-related diseases affecting the heart and circulation.

Vitamins are essential because they enable the body to make use of other nutrients. They provide the 'key' to many of the interlocking 'rooms' which form the human metabolic system. Until the beginning of the century they were unknown, and new discoveries are being made about them every day. Here's a brief guide to vitamins and their functions:

Vitamin A (fish liver oils, liver, eggs, dairy products, apricots and carrots) is essential for body growth, eye function, resistance to infection. It is soluble in fat, and can be stored in the liver, so two or three Vitamin A rich meals a week can be just as good as one a day. An overdose can be toxic, so don't drink unlimited carrot juice!

Vitamin B$_1$ (thiamine) (wheatgerm, yeast, wholemeal bread, lean meat) is essential for carbohydrate metabolism. Bread eaters should plump for wholemeal if possible, which helps nerves, digestion and the heart. It's soluble in water and cannot be stored, so get some every day.

Vitamin B$_2$ (riboflavin) (yeast, wheatgerm, liver, kidney, milk, cheese, meat) is good for skin, nails and hair and a deficiency leads to dull hair, split fingernails, itchy eyes. Luckily, this vitamin is likely to be sufficiently present in any diet which includes dairy products although it should be remembered that it can be destroyed by cooking and by light (a bottle of milk standing on a doorstep in bright sunshine can lose up to ten per cent of its riboflavin content every hour).

Nicotinic acid (yeast, wheatgerm, bread, liver, meat, fish) is for healthy skin, mucous membranes and the nervous system. It's less affected by heat and light than the other B vitamins although there are losses in cooking.

Vitamin B_6 (pyridoxin) (liver, kidneys) is vital for healthy skin and proper growth in children. There is some evidence that the contraceptive pill may cause vitamin B_6 depletion, and supplements are available for pill-takers.

Pantothenic acid (yeast, liver, beans) helps burn up fat from energy and is essential for fluid balance.

Folic acid (yeast, liver, milk, green vegetables) and *Vitamin B_{12}* (cynacocoblamin) (liver, meat) are both essential for healthy blood. Vitamin B_{12} is only in foods of animal origin, so Vegans – very strict vegetarians who eat absolutely no animal produce – can be deficient.

Vitamin C (ascorbic acid) (citrus fruits, green vegetables, potatoes) is for vitality, resistance to disease, and strengthening the connective tissues which make healthy bones, teeth and blood-vessels. It is soluble in water, and cooking losses can be *enormous* (up to 70 per cent for boiled green vegetables, for instance). It is not stored by the body, and many medical authorities feel that we need more vitamin C than we usually get, so it makes sense to 'top up' your daily intake from usual sources with some orange juice, especially if you intend to cut back on one fairly good source, potatoes, during a diet.

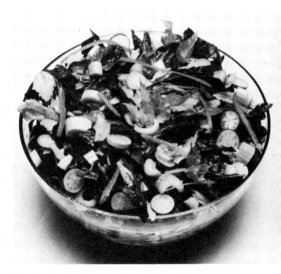

A mixed salad every day will boost your vitamin intake.

Vitamin D (cholecalciferol) (fish liver oils, eggs, milk, sunshine) is fascinating because it can be made by the body from sunshine. It regulates the calcium and phosphorous content of the body and is essential for the bone formation of children. Where the diet is low in vitamin D, and there is a lack of sunshine, rickets can occur. However, it can be stored by the liver, so a weekly serving is fine if you also get some exposure to the sun.

Vitamin E (tocopherol) (wheatgerm, wholegrains, wholewheat bread, nuts, vegetable oils) protects body tissues and keeps the blood circulating freely. It has been used to treat dry skin problems (externally) and as a treatment for heart disease (internally).

Vitamin K (dark green leafy vegetables, tomatoes, liver, carrot tops, soya bean oil) is essential to produce blood clotting, so step up your curly kale intake after cutting your hand badly or having an operation!

Minerals It's only now that the true importance of minerals in body metabolism is being realized. They help trigger off the action of vitamins, and play other important roles in keeping us healthy. The body contains about twenty minerals, eight needed in relatively large quantities and nine or more (we don't know yet!) are vital for normal metabolism in lesser amounts.

Iron (red meat, egg yolk, liver) is the top mineral for healthy ladies; it's been estimated that up to fifty per cent of women are iron-deficient.

Calcium (milk, cheese, yogurt) is vital for bone formation, even for adults – our bone formation is continually changing and being renewed – but especially in pregnant mums and children.

Other essential minerals include *iodine* (fish) for thyroid function, *zinc* (oysters, shellfish) for a healthy sex life, *sodium*, *potassium*, *chloride*, *magnesium* and *phosphorous*. To ensure a mineral rich diet it makes sense to eat widely, and to eat foods which are not over-processed or produced in artificial conditions, for we really do not know how much is lost by factory farming methods.

Fibre Although not strictly a nutrient, fibre is vital to help digestion and the passage of food through the body. It is particularly vital for slimmers because it adds bulk to the diet and makes it more satisfying. Fibre is, technically, the cellulose *and* hemicellulose present in plant tissues, the 'skeleton' of the plant. Most important sources are wholegrain cereals, starchy roots, pulses, vegetables and fruit. A good example of how fibre can work for slimmers is in comparing a high-fibre snack like an apple with a no-fibre snack like a cream cake. The apple takes some time to eat and digest and provides only 40 calories, the cream cake takes no time at all to eat and digest yet provides up to 300 calories! One high-fibre experiment conducted by medical nutrition experts involved feeding volunteers on unlimited quantities of baked potatoes and nothing else. All *lost* weight. Slimmers should remember that potatoes are not particularly high in calories, unless cooked in fat or eaten with butter and cream, and the skin is a useful source of fibre.

The five food groups

If you make sure that your daily diet includes foods from each of the groups listed below you will get your fair share of all the major nutrients. Keep referring to these food groups when planning your own diet and family menus.

Group 1 Meat of all kinds, poultry, offal, white and oily fish, shellfish, eggs. Main nutrients provided: protein, energy, fat, iron, vitamins B_1 and B_2, nicotinic acid.

Slimmers should choose something from this group each day, but cut off fat from meat and go for poultry or fish where possible as they are lower in calories. It's a good idea to eat liver or kidneys once a week.

Group 2 Dairy products: milk, cheese, cream, yogurt. Main nutrients provided: protein, energy, fat, calcium, vitamins A and B_2.

Slimmers should go easy on this group. Milk should be limited to half a pint or less, cheese should be strictly controlled as it is very high in calories. Yogurt is useful: nutritious, satisfying and good mixed with lemon juice as a salad dressing.

Group 3 Cereals: bread, flour, breakfast cereals, pasta, rice, peas, pulses, nuts. Main nutrients provided: energy, protein, carbohydrate, calcium, iron, Vitamins B_1 and B_2, nicotinic acid.

Slimmers will find wholemeal bread and pasta, unsweetened wholegrain cereals provide most nutrients and are very satisfying – a little goes a long way.

Group 4 Butter, margarine, cooking oils, fats. Main nutrients provided: energy, fat, vitamins A and D.

Slimmers beware: this group is calorie-loaded. You should limit butter and margarine intake to a scraping a day, and go very easy indeed on cooking oils and fats.

Group 5 Fruit and vegetables. Main nutrients provided: iron, vitamins A, B_1 and C, but vitamins can be lost in cooking.

Slimmers should let themselves go in this group, and eat as much as possible raw or lightly cooked to prevent nutrient loss. Try to make sure that you eat at least one piece of fresh fruit and one portion of salad vegetables daily.

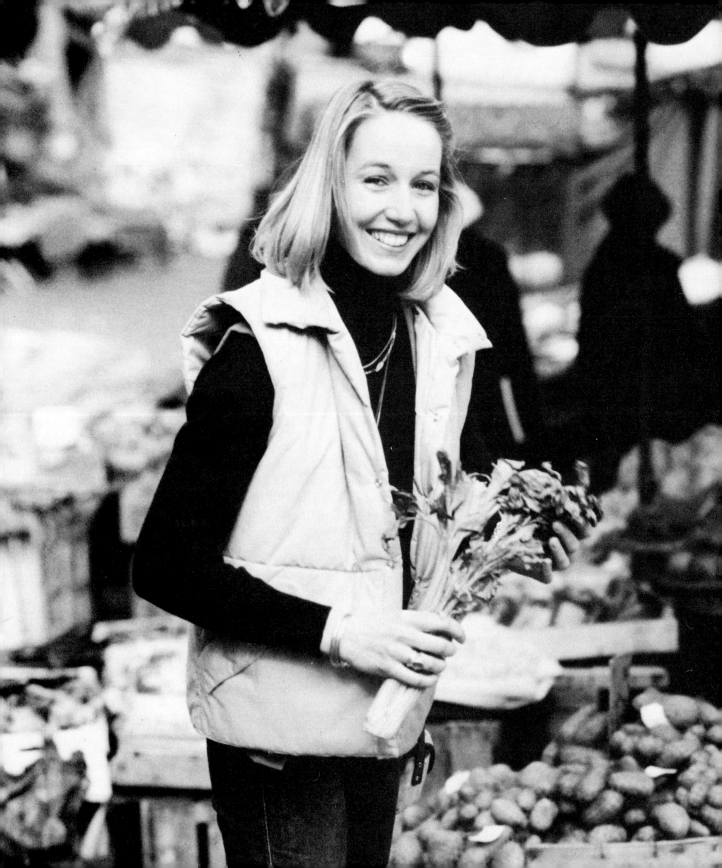

3 Dieting

Every new diet fad is greeted with shrieks of delight by people looking for a 'miracle' cure for the age-old problem of being overweight. Unfortunately, losing weight can be a highly complex thing – not strictly dependent on calorie intake or expenditure at all, but involved with such complex processes as metabolism and psychological hang-ups.

However, the basic rules remain – and it's worth recapping them here before talking more about the other, more complex side of the slimming coin.

Food unit measurement systems

What is a calorie? The amount of energy needed to heat a litre of water to just 1° centigrade. In the human body that energy is not required to heat water but to perform all the functions of the body, from breathing to running up a hill, from snoring to digesting food. The daily calorie requirement for adults varies according to age and the work they do, but for Ms Average it is 2100, and for Mr Average it is 2700. (He's usually a bit taller and broader, and more likely to be in an active job.) This figure, already suspect because it's 'average', is further confused because people's BMR (or Basal Metabolic Rate) varies too: this is the rate at which your body expels calories when at complete rest. Doctors measure this using a piece of apparatus called a Douglas bag. Expired air is collected over a period of time, then the total volume of gas is measured and the oxygen percentage calculated. Since there is a direct relationship between the volume of oxygen used and the number of calories expended by the body, the BMR can be calculated. It is hard luck if your BMR is very low; this means that you must follow a very low calorie diet indeed to lose weight, and try to 'rev up' your BMR, perhaps by increasing exercise or taking smaller meals more frequently.

Calorie-counting is a popular and fairly simple way of slimming – providing you make sure you follow a balanced diet *and* that you don't cheat when doing your calculations. It's essential to start by using a calorie chart to work out your *current* weekly food intake, then average it out on a daily basis. If you work out that your normal intake is 2000 calories daily, you can cut down to 1500 quite easily, having a weekly deficit of 350 or 460g (1lb) of body fat. You'd probably lose a bit of fluid too, so in two months you would shed over half a stone. If you wanted to lose weight more rapidly, then you could cut those calories to around 1000 or even 800 per day (but no less). Many diets are calculated on the basis of 1000 calories

Have fun choosing the very best market produce for your diet.

per day, which produces significant weight-loss in most people. If you follow such a diet faithfully you will almost certainly lose weight – unless you have a metabolic irregularity.

The big problem with calorie counting is *honesty*; if you don't write down that daily intake, you may forget things such as alcohol, or an extra slice of meat, which can throw out the calculations completely. However it is convenient for anyone who has to vary his or her diet for social reasons, or who needs flexibility. You do need a good knowledge of diet *balance* to work out your own calorie-counted diet – in order to get the very best foods. Products such as low-fat spreads, slimmers' soups, artificial sweeteners, diet drinks and no-calorie mixer drinks can be very helpful indeed, although I'm not keen on total meal replacement products. They tend to become boring and minimize your chances of eating good, wholesome, fresh foods.

Carbohydrate-counting Another way of counting calories, this system is based on the fact that high-carbohydrate foods like sugar and sweets are also high in calories, so if you restrict yourself to 50g of carbohydrate a day you will lose weight. Carbohydrate grams are usually expressed as units, one CU to 5g, so the arithmetic needed is much simpler. Each meal should consist of one carbohydrate-free food such as fish or meat, plus low-carbohydrate foods like green vegetables and salads. The problem is that people tend to overeat the carbohydrate-free foods on this kind of diet, and tot up lots of calories; there is also a problem with *alcohol*. Although spirits don't contain carbohydrate booze *is* calorie-loaded, so it has to be taken into account on this kind of diet. The best way of doing this is to give it a carbo-unit rating. The diet can also be expensive, since meat and fish are more expensive than, say, potatoes. But, if your maths are rotten, the diet can be terrific!

Fat-unit counting This is a new idea in diet calculation which uses the relatively new thinking about limiting fat intake for health. This method makes good sense, since fats are very high indeed in calories and can quite easily be restricted without the slimmer feeling deprived. Foods are given a fat-unit rating according to the quantity of fat they contain, and the number of units to be consumed is limited to 10 per day. It is really just another way of counting calories, and can be used very simply by slimmers who want to trim calories from their daily food intake: simply cut off all visible fat, stop eating butter on vegetables, and swap butter on bread for a low-fat spread such as Outline. Make sure you eat fish or white meat two or three times a week (less fat than red meat, which often contains quantities of hidden fat) and strictly *no* fatty cakes, puds or pastry. You'll find that lemon juice on its own makes a delicious substitute for oily salad dressings, and you can add it to *any* of the salads mentioned in the diets in this book. Fresh wholemeal bread is scrumptious without butter, and you'll begin to wonder why you swamped the taste of meat and vegetables with fat after you've tried grilling and light boiling (or, even better, steaming).

KiloJoules Since Britain joined the Common Market it has been decided to adopt this unit for energy from *all* sources, from the watts in a battery to the calories in a potato. The name comes from James Joule, an English physicist, who first evaluated the unit. KiloJoules will be the international unit in a few years' time, but the changeover will be gradual. They are not as yet commonly used to plan diets – perhaps quite fortunate for today's slimmers, for the kJ is equivalent to 4.184 calories and produces some rather unwieldy figures when you convert your daily calorie intake into the new units!

Serious dieting means weighing everything, even low-calorie fruit, not just guessing and grabbing!

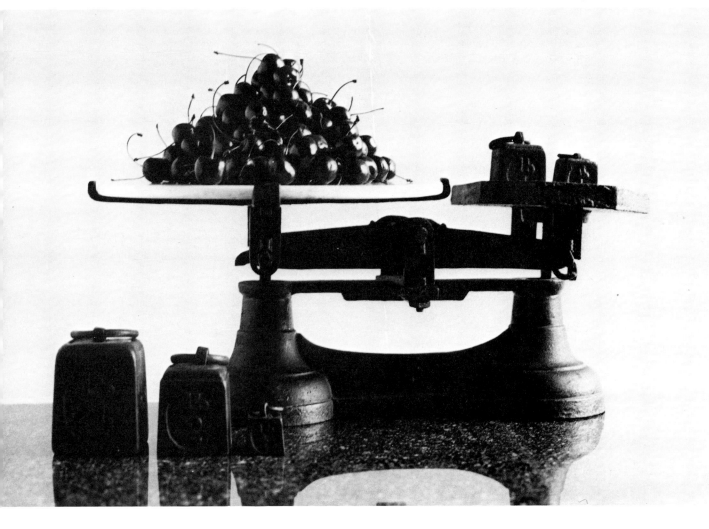

Calorie, kiloJoule and carbohydrate guide

Use this chart when planning your own diets. Stick to around 1000 calories (CAL), 4200 kiloJoules (KJ) or 10 carbohydrate units (CU – each one represents 5g of carbohydrates) per day, and select the foods which make up a balanced diet as described on page 26.

		CAL	KJ	CU
Apple	1 medium, raw	40	167	2
	1 large, baked	65	272	3
Apricots	2–3 raw	30	126	1½
	100g dried, stewed	25	104	1
	100g tinned	40	167	2
Artichokes, globe	100g boiled	15	63	1
Artichokes, Jerusalem	100g boiled	5	21	½
Aubergines	100g baked	15	63	1
Avocado	half	150	630	–
Bacon	2 back rashers, grilled	170	711	–
	2 streaky rashers, grilled	145	606	–
Banana	1 medium	65	272	3½
Beans	100g baked	100	420	2½
	100g broad, boiled	120	504	1½
	100g butter, boiled	94	395	2
	100g runner, boiled	20	164	½
Beef	100g corned	130	543	–
	100g mince	180	756	–
	100g steak, grilled	345	1442	–
	100g steak, stewed	230	961	–
Beetroot	1 boiled	25	104	1
Biscuits	2 small crackers	125	522	4
	2 small sweet	160	668	4½
Blackberries	100g raw	30	125	1½
	100g stewed	25	104	1
Blackcurrants	100g raw	30	125	1
	100g stewed	25	104	1
Bread	1 slice white	105	439	3
	1 slice wholemeal	65	272	2½
	1 slice calorie-reduced	33	138	1
	1 starch-reduced crispbread	24	100	½
Broccoli	100g boiled	15	63	–

		CAL	KJ	CU
Brussels sprouts	100g boiled	20	84	½
Cabbage	100g boiled	10	42	–
Cake	1 slice chocolate	350	1470	10
	1 slice fruit	250	1050	6
Carrots	100g boiled	25	104	1
Cauliflower	100g raw	16	68	–
	100g boiled	12	52	–
Celery	50g raw	14	117	–
Cereal	25g Cornflakes	100	418	4
	25g bran-based	99	414	4
	255 muesli	107	447	4
Cheese	50g Brie	190	794	–
	50g Camembert	175	731	–
	50g Cheddar	240	1003	–
	50g cottage	60	250	–
	50g Danish Blue	205	857	–
	50g Edam	175	731	–
	15g Parmesan	70	293	–
	50g Stilton	270	112	–
Cherries	100g raw	45	188	2½
Chicken	100g roast	168	–	
Chicory	100g raw	12	48	–
Cream	2 tbs single	60	251	–
	2 tbs double	130	543	–
Cucumber	½ medium	25	104	–
Currants	50g	140	602	7
Dates	5 raw	120	512	6
Duck	100g roast	355	1484	–
Eggs	large boiled	118	493	–
	small boiled	69	288	–
Fats	25g butter	225	940	–
	25g low-fat spread	100	418	–
	25g margarine	225	940	–
	1 tbs vegetable oil	120	604	–
Figs	3 raw	50	209	2
	100g dried, stewed	240	1008	4
Fish	100g white fish, grilled or baked	75	313	–
	100g oily fish, grilled or baked	100	418	–
	175g fried fish	390	1630	4
	3 fish fingers	145	606	2½

Food	Portion	CAL	KJ	CU
Fish	50g prawns	60	250	–
	50g smoked salmon	80	336	–
	50g tinned salmon	88	370	–
	50g tinned sardines	120	504	–
	50g tuna fish	120	504	–
Gooseberries	100g stewed	15	62	½
Grapefruit	half	15	62	½
Grapes	100g raw	70	292	3½
Ham	50g lean slices	175	731	–
Kidneys	75g braised	135	564	–
Lamb	100g chop, grilled	435	1818	–
	100g leg or shoulder, roast	304	1277	–
Leeks	100g boiled	30	125	1
Lemon	1 medium	15	62	1½
Lettuce	1 medium	15	62	–
Liver	100g grilled	170	711	–
Marrow	100g boiled	10	42	–
Mayonnaise	1 tbs	95	498	–
Melon	1 medium slice	15	62	1
Milk	1 pint (550ml) silver top	370	1554	5½
	1 pint skimmed or low-fat powdered	200	840	2½
Mushrooms	50g grilled	4	17	–
Nuts	50g almonds	340	1421	½
	50g Brazil	365	1526	½
	50g cashew	320	1344	½
	50g chestnuts	100	418	4
	50g salted peanuts	365	1526	1
	50g walnuts	310	1296	½
Olives	25g tinned	24	100	
Onion	50g raw	14	59	–
	50g boiled	10	42	–
Orange	1 medium	40	167	2
Orange, mandarin	100g tinned	70	292	3½
Parsnips	100g boiled	65	272	3
Pasta	100g boiled	115	481	5
Pastry	25g flaky	165	690	2½
	25g shortcrust	155	648	3
Peaches	1 medium	35	146	2
	100g tinned	90	376	5
Pears	1 medium	35	146	2
	100g tinned	90	376	5
Peas	100g boiled	15	63	1
Peppers	1 medium, green or red	30	125	1
Pineapple	1 slice raw	25	104	1½
	100g tinned	90	378	3

Food	Portion	CAL	KJ	CU
Plums	4 raw	60	248	4
	100g stewed	25	104	1
Pork	100g chop, grilled	510	2132	–
	100g leg or loin, roast	360	1505	–
Potatoes	1 medium baked	175	731	8
	100g chips	330	1379	8
	100g boiled	92	386	7
Prunes	100g dried, stewed	140	585	7
Pulses	100g dried, boiled	110	480	4
Radishes	50g raw	10	42	–
Raspberries	100g raw or stewed	30	126	1
Rhubarb	100g stewed	4	17	–
Rice	100g boiled	140	585	7
Sausages	2 grilled	385	1609	–
Soups	half-pint (275ml), consommé	85	357	–
	half-pint minestrone	150	640	1
	half-pint tinned tomato	175	725	2
Spinach	100g boiled	30	125	–
Spring greens	100g boiled	10	42	–
Strawberries	100g raw	30	125	1
Sweetcorn	100g boiled	100	418	4
Tangerines	2 medium	28	117	1
Tomatoes	2 medium raw	16	66	–
	100g tinned	12	50	–
Turkey	100g roast	225	940	–
Turnips	100g boiled	10	42	½
Veal	100g fried escalope	245	1024	1
Watercress	50g	10	42	3
Yogurt	1 small carton, plain	75	313	2
Beer	1 pint (550ml) brown ale	160	669	8
	1 pint draught bitter	180	752	8½
	1 pint draught mild	140	585	7
	1 pint lager	150	627	7½
	1 pint pale ale	180	752	9
	1 pint stout	200	836	10½
Brandy	1 pub measure	75	313	3
Cider	half-pint (275ml) dry	100	418	5
	half-pint sweet	120	502	6
Gin	1 pub measure	55	229	2½
Sherry	1 pub measure dry	55	229	3
	1 pub measure sweet	65	271	3½
Port	1 pub measure	75	313	3
Vermouth	1 pub measure dry	55	229	3
Whisky	1 pub measure	60	250	–
Wine	1 glass dry	90	376	4
	1 glass sweet	115	480	5

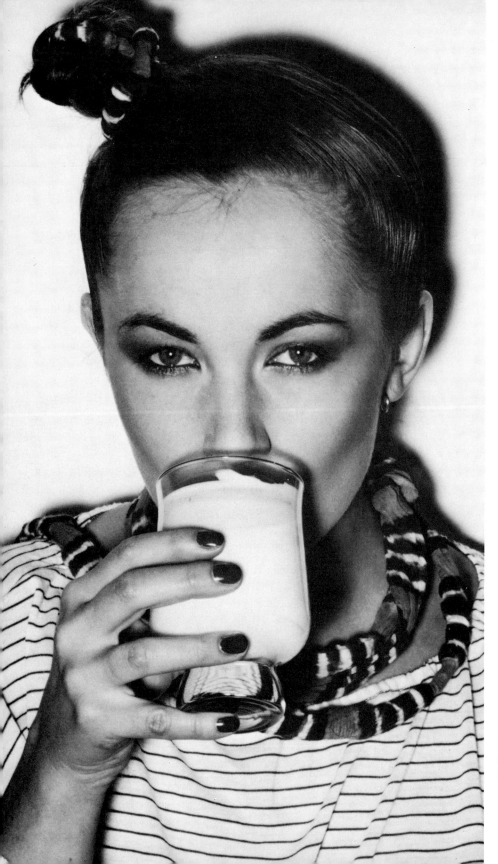

In a hurry? *Drink* your breakfast! A nutritious milkshake is a delicious start to the day.

You and your diet

Before you start Take into consideration your lifestyle, your food likes and dislikes, family commitments and budget before going on a diet. Generally speaking, you can tailor your present diet with an overall reduction, using any of the food unit measurement systems in the chart on the previous pages. Or you can try any one of the specialist diets in the next section. If you have a lot of weight to lose, choose a diet which allows a flexible eating pattern; it's unrealistic to envisage staying on a *strict* regime for weeks on end, although perfectly possible for a few days or a week. All the diets included here are designed to help establish good eating habits for the future; there are foods which may be unusual to you, and dishes with interesting texture and tastes. Aim to make your diet a culinary experience as well as a way of slimming – that way it will be fun and less of a hardship.

It's unfair, but true, that men usually have less problem sticking to a diet and losing weight than women. One American doctor, Barbara Edelstein, who practises in Connecticut and specializes in female slimming problems, maintains that men lose weight almost twice as fast as women. The reason? A woman's body is naturally composed of a higher proportion of fat to muscle tissue than a man's, and muscle mass burns five more calories per pound to maintain itself than fat or connective tissue.

Women are further discriminated against by their monthly hormonal cycle. During the pre-menstrual period we are more likely to crave sweets (especially chocolate), can be up to five or six pounds heavier from water retention, and may feel depressed; all of which can combine to put us right off dieting. Strategy? During this time, reduce your intake of salt and avoid soups, but drink water. It sounds crazy, but plain old water has a diuretic effect and actually expels fluid from your body via the kidneys. Don't weigh yourself until your period begins. If you are on the pill, you may experience a small weight-gain – if it's large, and you really haven't been eating more, you should consult your doctor immediately. Some women report that the newer mini-pills don't produce a significant weight-gain.

What about the menopause? As if female changes *before* the menopause weren't bad enough, the menopause conspires to do the nasty on slimmer women. Fat women have usually gained as much weight as they are going to by this time, but the mechanism of weight-gain in menopause appears to be the enlargement of fat cells. You really do need to decrease your daily calorie intake by 5 per cent for every five years after the age of forty. Sorry!

Even though they may not be as obvious as the feminine ones, men do experience slimming hazards in their own right. Hazard number one: boozing. Lager is a killer for inflating your tums, so stick to half-pints and make them *last*. If your loved ones adore piling food on your plate (and women are often guilty of expressing love for their men in terms of carbohydrate!) be firm about the fact that you are *slimming*. Encourage your lover to make you amazingly sexy salads instead of suet puds. Men, too, need to decrease their daily calorie intake after forty (earlier if you are the lazy type). Unfairly, it's often the most athletic men who suffer most from middle-age spread; once you give up football or rugby the pounds pile on. Don't forget that squash or badminton can be played all year round, and you don't have to be in your twenties to be good at either.

Successful dieting Having made the decision to diet, do stick to it, however short the period. To help you stay the course, here are a few hints:

Incentive is vital. Keep a worthwhile goal in mind as you slim – a shopping spree, a holiday or other treat, or someone you want to impress . . . don't make the prize at the end of the dieting rainbow edible! If your loved ones are encouraging, great – if not, try to resist their offers of sweets, cakes and other temptations. Remember, their motives may be suspect – maybe you're more useful as you are! You've got to be very determined yet cheerfully polite to diet-detractors. No rows, just be quiet, calm and sure.

Group therapy is fun with the ones you love, but if that isn't possible get support from friends or colleagues with the same intention in mind; join a group such as Weight Watchers or a slimming club. Many women have found tremendous help within one of the feminist-orientated groups which help you cope with the psychological problems attached to losing weight. If you are the earth mother type, who habitually stuffs herself with food, or think you may be using food as a substitute for other comforts, head straight for one of these groups (see list on page 110). They'll help you sort out your head first, body later.

Keep a diary of the foods you eat. This is particularly vital if you're following a calorie, carbohydrate or fat-unit controlled diet, with comments about *how you felt* when you eat. Behaviour therapy such as this can help you assess the associations food has for you, and how to cope with them. Note where you eat, when you eat, and keep a weekly weight record. Use the diary to note possible hazards later; parties, outings and dire events such as exams, a driving test, or a work conference which could send you screaming for a cream bun! On those days, beat the eating trap by taking your food with you; apple, orange, or raw vegetables. When nerves take over, you won't be at the mercy of the corner cake shop or hamburger joint!

Watch out for hunger traps such as driving and shopping. On a long-distance drive, avert temptation by packing a picnic and keeping some no-calorie chewing gum and fresh fruit in the car. It's all too easy to pull over and pick up a fast food snack. Don't do it! Never go shopping on an empty stomach. Eat before you do the family shopping, and before you go out to shop at lunchtime. Wear perfume all the time to make you less vulnerable to food smells. Avoid shops which you know are tempting: fish and chip shops, delicatessens, bakers' shops, sweetshops. Don't rush into a supermarket if you only want vegetables, instead choose a green-grocer's or street market where the produce may be cheaper and fresher, and where you won't be faced with shelves of biscuits and sweets at the check-out counter. There is no reason why shopping shouldn't be a pleasure – *the* perfect green pepper, a delicious display of apples, good fresh meat – and why not grab some flowers to make your table look good?

Cooking can be dangerous! If you have to produce cakes and puds for the rest of the family, do it on a full stomach. But I really don't think it's unreasonable to get them to do their own baking while you are slimming, or better still, to get them to slim with you. If you have to prepare meals for young children give them just enough, don't prepare extra for *you* to finish up. Older kids are usually delighted to do their own thing; I recently bought my eleven-year-old son a sandwich-toasting machine so he can prepare his own tea while I stay out of the kitchen! Serve each meal as if it were a banquet, with pretty tablecloth, cutlery, glasses, and all the trimmings. If you're dishing up puds and chips for non-slimmers, keep the portions small so there really isn't enough for you.

Eating should be done slowly, chewing each mouthful thoroughly. Don't bolt your food; if you do your tum doesn't really get a chance to send 'full up' signals to your brain before another lot of food comes flying down. Experiments with slimmers have shown that the slower form of eating can help them feel much more satisfied on less food. Think of the Japanese (eat out at a Japanese restaurant every night, if you can afford it, for the perfect diet) who prepare very small, delicate meals and eat them slowly and lovingly! Try to leave *something* on your plate, even it it's only a lettuce leaf. Fatties have often been conditioned to consume everything in front of them, whether they are hungry or not. Beat that one by training *yourself* to stop when you've had enough.

One word of warning: don't embark on a *drastic* slimming diet while recuperating from an operation, having a baby, or after a serious emotional upset. Instead, concentrate on improving the quality of your diet (look again at the Five Food Groups on page 26) and wait until you feel physically and mentally strong again.

The body clock diet

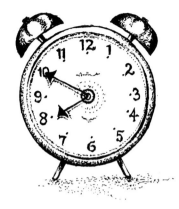

Ever thought of your body as a *clock*? It keeps time just as efficiently as the latest quartz alarm, starting slowly in the morning, rising to a peak of efficiency during the day, slowing down again at night. You should be able to tell the time by your body, monitoring the little signs that indicate that it's early in the day, or late.

Slimming doctors in America have harnessed this aspect of our body rhythm to produce some remarkable results with obese patients. They maintain that the body is geared to deal with the *maximum number* of calories early in the day; a bumper breakfast, substantial lunch and light evening meal. Experiments at the University of Minnesota Medical School showed that slimmers who use this pattern lose weight quickly and easily; if they eat the same number of calories later in the day, it's far harder to lose weight.

This one-week diet follows these 'body clock' principles, with over *half* the daily calorie total consumed before the afternoon. Breakfast-haters should have one of the high-calorie liquid breakfasts on page 39 instead of tucking into a large spread. Benefits? As well as helping you to lose weight faster, the diet will make you feel efficient and bright at work and help you to avoid that bloated mid-evening feeling. Use the time you are on the diet to take up some kind of evening activity, keep-fit classes for instance, and plan your breakfast the night before to avoid rushing in the morning.

Daily Allowances One-third pint whole milk for use in tea and coffee. Use only low-calorie spreads on bread, no butter.

Day 1

Breakfast Unsweetened orange juice; small bowl muesli; 2 slices wholemeal toast; 1 poached egg.

Lunch Grilled chicken leg; large portion salad; 1 slice wholemeal bread; 1 banana.

Supper 1 bowl calorie-reduced soup; 1 crispbread; fresh fruit salad with natural yogurt.

Day 2

Breakfast Small tin baked beans on 1 slice wholemeal toast topped with a little grated cheese; 1 pear; 1 fruit yogurt.

Lunch Hamburger without bun; 1 baked potato; 1 orange.

Supper 2 slices cold chicken; a green salad.

Day 3

Breakfast 1 slice of melon; 2 lean bacon rashers and 2 tomatoes grilled; 1 slice wholemeal toast; 1 tbs sweetcorn.

Lunch Grilled fish (large portion); boiled broccoli or spinach; 1 boiled potato; 1 apple.

Supper 1 poached egg on 1 slice wholemeal toast; a green salad.

Day 4

Breakfast Unsweetened grapefruit juice; 1 slice ham on 1 slice toast, topped with sliced tomato and cheese and browned under the grill; 1 orange.

Lunch 1 bowl calorie-reduced soup; 1 slice wholemeal bread; 50g well-drained tuna; a mixed salad.

Supper Large portion fresh fruit salad with natural yogurt.

Day 5

Breakfast Tomato juice; 1 grilled kipper; 1 slice wholemeal bread; 1 pear.

Lunch 2 slices ham; potato salad with Slender Mayonnaise (see page 61); lettuce and cucumber; 1 slice wholemeal bread.

Supper Clear soup; 1 boiled egg; 1 slice wholemeal bread; 1 orange.

Day 6

Breakfast Grated carrot and cucumber salad with lemon-juice dressing; 2 scrambled eggs on 1 slice wholemeal toast; 2 grilled tomatoes.

Lunch A salad of 2 tbs cottage cheese on 2 well-drained tinned pineapple rings with lettuce, tomatoes, chopped apple, celery, watercress; 1 slice wholemeal bread; 1 fruit yogurt.

Supper 1 bowl calorie-reduced soup; 1 slice wholemeal bread with a one-inch cube hard cheese.

Day 7

Breakfast Kedgeree made with rice, smoked fish and peas; unsweetened orange juice.

Lunch 2 slices lean roast meat; 100g green beans or broccoli; 1 boiled potato; baked apple with raisins.

Supper Large portion fresh fruit salad; 1 slice wholemeal bread.

Liquid breakfasts

1 Blend 1 banana, 1 carton natural yogurt and a dash of lemon juice. Dilute to taste with milk from allowance.

2 Blend small glass tomato juice, 1 egg, 1 carton natural yogurt with dash of lemon juice and Worcestershire sauce.

3 Squeeze two oranges and blend with 1 orange-flavoured yogurt and the juice of half a lemon. Stir in 1 tbs mixed nuts and 1 tsp honey. Eat with a spoon!

The avocado diet

Avocados are a good source of minerals and vitamins which can help keep you feeling, and looking, good. Although they are not particularly low in calories (about 160 for a medium-sized half avocado) they are very satisfying and convenient to eat. They contain potassium, sodium, magnesium, phosphorus, calcium and a little iron. They are rich in folic acid and also contain vitamin C, some protein, fat and carbohydrate.

Great beauties have used the flesh and skin of the avocado for centuries; the natural oils contained in the flesh make a super face-pack (you

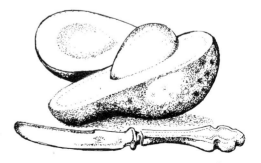

can whizz it up in the blender with egg-yolk or thick yogurt), and the used skins can be rubbed on hard skin (elbows, knees) to help soften it.

Try this short diet when you want to feel pampered (it's a favourite with screen beauties like Farah Fawcett and Jackie Bissett) and when avocados are widely available.

Daily allowances One-third pint milk for use in tea or coffee; 1 slice wholemeal bread. Unlimited mineral water or diet soft drinks.

Day 1

Breakfast Peel and slice half an avocado; brush with lemon juice. Peel 1 orange and divide into segments. Arrange the fruit on a plate and top with 50g cottage cheese.

Lunch Blend half an avocado with half a small carton low-fat natural yogurt, a squeeze of lemon juice and seasonings. Serve with crudités – raw green pepper, celery, carrot and cauliflower.

Supper Peel, dice and toss half an avocado in lemon juice. Mix with 100g diced roast chicken and half a grapefruit peeled and divided into segments. Serve on a bed of chinese cabbage.

Day 2

Breakfast Blend half an avocado with a squeeze of lemon juice, seasonings and 50g low-fat soft cheese. Spread on 2 crisp-breads.

Lunch Peel and dice half an avocado; toss in lemon juice. Mix with 75g diced Edam cheese and 12 seeded grapes. Serve on a bed of lettuce.

Supper Make a salad of 1 tomato and half a peeled and sliced avocado. Serve with 150g grilled plaice fillet, sprinkled with lemon juice and seasoning.

Day 3

Breakfast Blend half an avocado with 1 carton low-fat natural yogurt and a small glass of apple juice.

Lunch Peel and dice half an avocado. Mix with 50g chopped raw sprouts and 75g diced Camembert. Top with half a small carton seasoned low-fat natural yogurt.

Supper Remove the yolks from 2 halved hard-boiled eggs and mash with half an avocado, a squeeze of lemon juice, half a carton of low-fat natural yogurt and seasoning. Pile the mixture into the cavity of egg whites and serve with sliced tomatoes.

Day 4

Breakfast Blend 1 hard-boiled egg with half an avocado, lemon juice, seasoning and 1 tbs tomato juice. Spread on 2 crispbreads.

Lunch Peel and slice half an avocado, brush with lemon juice, and lay it on 2 thin slices of tongue. Cover with 50g celery cut into strips and 1 chopped tomato. Serve with watercress.

Supper Avocado Stuffed Pepper (see page 57).

Breakfast Blend half an avocado with a squeeze of lemon juice, half a carton of low-fat natural yogurt and a small glass of tomato juice.

Lunch Slice half an avocado, brush with lemon juice and place on a bed of finely chopped raw cabbage. Top with 100g seasoned cottage cheese with chives.

Supper Peel and dice half an avocado; core and dice 1 apple. Toss both in lemon juice and mix with 100g prawns and 25g chopped celery. Decorate with a few toasted almond flakes.

The pasta diet

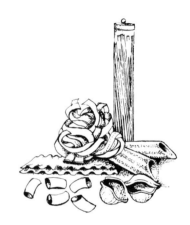

Just to prove that slimming isn't necessarily all about giving up the foods you love most, here's a diet based on what is usually considered a 'sinful' dish for slimmers – pasta (it contains about 70 per cent carbohydrate, 13 per cent protein, some fibre, and a little fat). In fact, poor old pasta isn't really calorie-loaded at all – a generous 50g raw portion works out at 208 calories when cooked – but the *sauces* which go with it are often very fattening indeed. So the way to use spaghetti, tagliatelle, lasagne and the other delicious varieties of pasta in your slimming programme is to eat them with *low*-calorie sauces and salads.

For example, take your basic 208 calorie pasta portion; add a knob or two of butter, some bolognaise sauce and a sprinkling of cheese, and you can quickly push up the calorie total to around 700. If instead you add a few chopped prawns, fresh tomato purée, lemon juice and herbs, the meal amounts to only 350 calories and is still rich in minerals and vitamins with a respectable amount of protein. The secret is to limit the *fat*; don't toss your pasta in oil, butter or cream . . . instead follow the guidelines set out in the diet below. The extras are for manual workers, very active women or greedy children!

Daily allowances Half a pint low-fat milk for use in tea or coffee. Unlimited water, mineral water, lemon tea, black coffee.

Breakfast Every day have one of the following 300-calorie breakfasts:
• 1 slice melon; 1 poached egg on 1 slice wholemeal toast; small glass grapefruit or orange juice; tea or coffee.
• Half grapefruit; 2 lean rashers of bacon, grilled; 50g mushrooms grilled; 1 tomato grilled; 1 small slice wholemeal bread topped with a scraping of butter; black coffee or lemon tea.
• 50g pre-cooked macaroni tossed with 1 tbs natural yogurt and orange segments; the juice of a whole orange topped up with a little water; tea or coffee.
• Small tin spaghetti in tomato sauce or spaghetti rings on small slice wholemeal toast (no butter) topped with 1 sliced tomato; 1 apple; tea or coffee.

- Fruit yogurt; 1 starch-reduced crispbread; 25g Edam cheese; small glass orange juice; black coffee or lemon tea.
- 50g cold, pre-cooked pasta mini shells mixed with 1 tbs sweetcorn, chopped red pimento and 1 dsp low-calorie salad dressing; tea or coffee.
- 25g muesli with a little milk and stewed rhubarb; 1 slice lean ham; large glass grapefruit juice; black coffee or lemon tea.
- 50g pre-cooked short cut macaroni mixed with chopped ½ green pepper, 1 slice lean ham and 1 dsp low-calorie mayonnaise; tea or coffee.

Day 1

Lunch Pasta and Chicken Salad (see page 61).
1 orange.

Supper Italian Vegetable Soup (see page 57); 150g haddock fillet grilled with lemon juice and chives; green beans or cauliflower.

Extras Pasta portion; 1 slice wholewheat bread.
1 pint bitter or 2 glasses dry wine.

Day 2

Lunch 1 hard-boiled egg; 1 slice wholewheat bread; cheese spread triangle.
1 apple and 1 banana.

Supper 50g spaghetti with Tomato Sauce (see page 61) mixed with 50g chopped prawns and a squeeze of lemon juice; a mixed salad.
100g strawberries.

Extras Pasta portion and sauce; 50g prawns.
Half-pint bitter or 1 glass dry wine.

Day 3

Lunch 1 bowl Italian Vegetable Soup (see page 57); 25g slice corned beef with 1 slice wholemeal bread.

Supper 50g cold pasta shells tossed in lemon juice and chopped mint and mixed with diced cucumber, sliced mushrooms, watercress and 25g drained tuna.
100g raspberries.

Extras 25g tuna; 1 carton natural yogurt; 1 slice wholewheat bread.
1 pint bitter or 2 glasses dry wine.

Day 4

Lunch Open sandwich with 25g tuna, chopped spring onion, lettuce, 1 tsp lemon juice, 2 tsp Slender Mayonnaise (see page 61); 1 slice wholemeal bread.
1 orange.

Supper Baked or grilled chicken drumstick; small can spaghetti rings; 75g peas.
1 apple.

Extras Jacket potato; small pat butter; fruit yogurt.
Half-pint bitter or 1 glass dry wine.

Day 5

Lunch   25g small pasta shells or noodles cooked in 1 tin calorie-reduced chicken soup; 1 slice wholemeal bread; 1 cheese spread triangle; 1 tomato.

Supper   100g Haddock Bake (see page 59); 50g large pasta shells; a green salad.
1 baked apple.

Extras   Pasta portion; 1 slice wholewheat bread.
1 pint bitter or 2 glasses dry wine.

Day 6

Lunch   Melon Picnic (see page 58).

Supper   50g fettuccine with 1 serving Tomato Sauce; 25g grated Edam cheese.
1 pear.

Extras   Wholemeal sandwich with yeast extract, watercress and tomato; 2 rashers well-grilled back bacon.
1 pint bitter or 2 glasses dry wine.

Day 7

Lunch   2 slices lean roast beef; 100g portion cauliflower; 50g large pasta shells with parsley and lemon juice.
2 canned pineapple rings, drained.

Supper   1 bowl calorie-reduced minestrone; 1 slice wholemeal bread.
1 fruit yogurt.

Extras   1 slice roast beef; 1 slice wholemeal bread; 50g large pasta shells.
Half-pint bitter or 1 glass dry wine.

Day 8

Lunch   Pasta and Chicken Salad (see page 61).
1 orange.

Supper   Yogurt Stroganoff (see page 60); a green salad.

Extras   2 slices wholemeal bread sandwiched with cheese triangle; 1 large or two small potatoes.
Half-pint bitter or 1 glass dry wine.

Day 9

Lunch   1 bowl Italian Vegetable Soup; 1 slice wholemeal bread.
1 orange.

Supper   50g spaghetti, tagliatelle or pasta shapes with Tomato Sauce and 25g grated Edam cheese.

Extras   Spaghetti portion and sauce.
Half-pint bitter or 1 glass dry wine.

Day 10

Lunch   Open sandwich of 25g chicken on 1 slice wholemeal bread plus lettuce and tomato.
1 banana.

Supper   Baked Fish with Pasta (see page 59); 2 sliced tomatoes tossed in lemon juice with herbs and salt.

Extras   1 slice wholemeal bread and scraping of butter; 1 fruit yogurt. Half-pint bitter or 1 glass dry wine.

Day 11

Lunch   Wholewheat sandwich made with 1 slice lean ham, lettuce and cucumber.
1 apple.

Supper   Mexican Casserole (see page 60); a green salad.

Extras   Mexican Casserole portion.
Half-pint beer or 1 glass dry wine.

Day 12

Lunch   Melon Picnic (see page 58).

Supper   50g macaroni and cheese sauce made with 25g Edam.
Fresh fruit salad.

Extras   Small lamb chop, well grilled.
1 pint bitter or 2 glasses dry wine.

Day 13

Lunch   1 bowl calorie-reduced minestrone; 1 slice wholewheat bread with cheese spread triangle.

Supper   Chicken Lasagne (see page 59); a green salad.

Extras   Extra portion lasagne.
Half-pint bitter or 1 glass dry wine.

Day 14

Lunch   50g lean roast pork; boiled cabbage and broccoli; 50g any pasta shape.

Supper   1 bowl Italian Vegetable Soup; 1 slice wholewheat bread.

Extras   50g roast pork; 1 fruit yogurt.
Half-pint bitter or 1 glass dry wine.

The wine and dine diet

This is just the kind of self-indulgence you need if you haven't the time for a holiday this year – and the results are marvellous. Treats like lemon sole, guinea-fowl, smoked salmon and Steak Tartare will be relished by the most jaded palates, *and* there's a booze allowance. There are loads of vegetables in this diet, and do remember to cook them very lightly to keep as much of their nutritional value as possible.

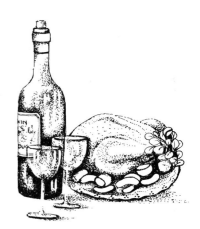

Daily allowances Half a pint whole milk or 1 pint skimmed milk in tea or coffee or alone. 1 glass spirits (but use low-calorie tonic or fizzies) or 2 glasses wine.

Breakfast Start every day with half a grapefruit or fresh orange or lemon juice topped up with water, and then have one of the following:
• 1 lean rasher bacon, 50g each tomatoes and mushrooms grilled.

- 1 egg, boiled, baked or poached, with 1 thin slice wholemeal bread and a little butter.
- 1 small (150g) piece of fish, grilled or poached, and 1 apple, pear or peach.
- Scrambled eggs (2) on 1 slice wholemeal bread.
- 100g kidneys or 75g liver, 100g tomatoes, grilled.

Day 1

Lunch 50g smoked salmon with sprigs of watercress and a slice of lemon; 1 thin slice wholemeal bread and a little butter.
1 sliced fresh pear with 25g Edam, chopped and seasoned with black pepper.

Supper Half a tin chilled consommé garnished with finely sliced cucumber and chives.
Quarter chicken rubbed with garlic and lemon juice and grilled; 50g button mushrooms and 50g tomatoes sprinkled with oregano and grilled; boiled French beans.
2 leaves chicory, 1 radish and 25g Edam.

Day 2

Lunch Salad of 50g diced cucumber, 50g tomatoes, 50g cubed Edam, 1 black olive, finely sliced raw onion, seasoned with coriander, black pepper and lemon juice.
1 sliced fresh orange sprinkled with cloves, cinnamon and chopped fresh mint.

Supper 100g prawns with lemon juice; 1 slice toast and a little butter.
Grilled calves liver with tarragon; boiled broccoli.
2 fresh passion-fruit sliced open and served with 1 tsp natural yogurt on each half.

Day 3

Lunch Cheese and Broccoli Flan (see page 58); salad of 100g tomatoes with chopped fresh basil, black pepper and lemon juice.
100g fresh raspberries, 1 tbs single cream and a sprig of mint.

Supper 175g lemon sole (on the bone) grilled with 25g Edam cheese; 100g raw salsify or celery; boiled spinach.
1 carton natural yogurt and 6 black cherries.

Day 4

Lunch Cheese and tomato omelette made with 2 eggs, 15g Edam and 1 dsp chopped parsley; green salad tossed in lemon juice.
1 peach.

Supper 50g raw mushrooms mixed with half a carton natural yogurt, lemon juice and black pepper.
150g roast guinea-fowl; boiled spinach; raw cauliflower sprigs.
100g fresh apricots.

Day 5

Lunch 1 hard-boiled egg halved, yolks chopped with 25g prawns and put back into the egg whites, topped with Edam and grilled gently; 2 sticks celery. 2 greengages.

Supper   Cucumber and mint soup made by liquidizing half a carton natural yogurt, half a cucumber, 2 sprigs of mint and seasoning. Serve chilled.
100g grilled steak; a mixed salad.
75g blackberries with 1 tbs single cream.

Day 6
Lunch   1 poached egg on a bed of lightly cooked spring greens (about 150g).
1 orange.

Supper   1 thin slice Parma ham with 1 slice melon, seasoned with ginger.
Steak Tartare made with 75g minced beef fillet, 1 beaten egg, chopped capers, onion, parsley and seasoning; a salad of 150g sliced tomatoes.
Fresh fruit salad.

Day 7
Lunch   50g roast lamb with mint sauce; boiled courgettes and runner beans.
25g Edam with 3 spring onions; 1 apple.

Supper   1 slice quiche made with leeks or asparagus (see Cheese and Broccoli Flan recipe on page 58 for method); lettuce and herb salad.
1 sliced orange mixed with 50g loganberries flavoured with cloves.

The vitamin A diet

This is a seven-day diet that takes in all the good things needed by the eye and brain – it gives a general feeling of well-being too, and I recommend it for anyone working for exams or any project requiring long hours of close paperwork or handwork.

Eyes need vitamin A, but mild deficiencies in it are common. The first symptom is difficulty in seeing in the dark; if you're a driver you can test your vitamin A level quite easily. If your ocular fluid contains enough of it you will be able to see again almost immediately after passing cars with headlamps full on, but if you're deficient you'll be blinded! Other symptoms include tiredness after watching television, headaches and sensitivity to bright light during the day. People who work under fluorescent light, and those who work in dim light, requiring good night vision, are particularly in need of adequate supplies of vitamin A, as are photographers, anyone spending time on snowy ski-slopes or glaring white sand, and office and factory workers.

Vitamin B_2 (riboflavin) is also vital for your eyes. Early symptoms of

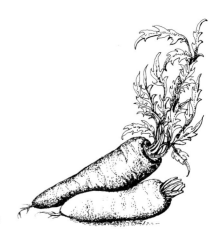

deficiency are similar to those for vitamin A deficiency, but with the added bonus of sore and bloodshot eyes. When vitamin B_2 supplies are inadequate, the body cannot renew the cells in the cornea (the tissue covering the eye) and tiny blood-vessels are formed.

Your eyes contain more vitamin C than any other part of the body, except the endocrine glands; it keeps the capillary walls and connective tissue of the eye system healthy. Unfortunately many people fail to take in enough vitamin C (especially men, who are not noted for their love of citrus fruits and green vegetables) although it is really easy to absorb it through a glass of orange juice or a grapefruit for breakfast every day.

Steer clear of blood-vessel-distending booze during the week you follow this diet, but drink lots of still mineral water, Evian for instance. Don't indulge in lots of sugary fizzy drinks.

Daily allowance Half a pint whole milk for use in tea or coffee.

Breakfasts A large glass of unsweetened orange juice and a cup of tea or coffee with milk (but no sugar) and *one* of the following:
• Muesli with apricots (fresh or dried) or peaches and milk.
• Scrambled eggs (2) mixed with chopped green pepper, tomato and chives on 1 slice wholemeal toast.
• Mixed grill of 1 small piece liver, 1 kidney and 50g mushrooms, with watercress and 1 slice wholemeal toast.

Lunches Choose one each day:
• A 50g piece of cheese and a mixed salad, including grated carrot.
• Grilled white fish (100g) with lemon wedge and parsley; a green salad.
• Sardines (4) on 1 slice wholemeal toast with lemon wedge and parsley.
• Herb omelette (2 eggs) with boiled spinach or green salad.
• 2 thin slices ham with a mixed salad.
• The Raw Dip: scrub crudités (raw carrot, cauliflower, celery, etc.) and make a dip with half a small carton cottage cheese, grated onion, chopped green or red pepper, lemon juice and seasoning. For the office, prepare this the night before and pack the crudités and dip in separate air-tight containers.

Suppers Choose one each day, but you must have liver *twice*. Each supper should be accompanied by 1 slice wholemeal bread with a scraping of butter:
• Grilled mackerel stuffed with mushrooms and capers; a salad of raw carrot and mushrooms.
• Braised liver (100g) with orange slices and boiled spinach.
• Curried liver (100g) with brown rice and a green salad.
• Grilled liver (100g) with boiled carrots and potatoes (in their skins).
• Pork chop with stewed apricots and brown rice; tomato and mushroom salad.

- Cold lean meat with a mixed salad (have a good selection of raw green vegetables and grated carrot).
- Cauliflower cheese (made with 25g Edam); carrots cooked in orange juice with a little seasoning and potatoes boiled in their skins.

The high fibre diet

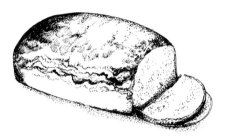

Fibre is the 'scaffolding' that supports plant cells; it helps prevent such diseases as diverticulitis and bowel cancer, and those affecting the heart and gall-bladder. It can also be helpful for slimmers, in several important ways. One: fibre-rich foods are more satisfying than low-fibre foods (compare eating an apple with a slice of cream cake). Two: there is evidence that fibre-eaters excrete more fat in their stools than those on a low-fibre diet. Three: it helps beat constipation, often a big problem for fatties!

Try this diet for a week if you're fed up with feeling hungry on ordinary low-calorie diets, or if you feel that fibre could help with other health problems as well as your wobbly waistline. Warning: don't kid yourself that you are 'slimming' if you gorge on wholemeal bread, brown rice and naughty nuts from the health food shop. Some fibre-rich foods need controlling carefully if you want to lose weight.

Daily allowances Half a pint fresh whole milk; 3 slices wholemeal bread with low-fat spread. Drink half a pint of fibre-rich Guinness or two glasses of white wine, and plenty of water to encourage elimination.

Day 1
Breakfast	Fresh fruit salad (use a mixture of fruits and leave the skins *on* where possible) topped with one carton natural yogurt and lemon juice; slice of bread from allowance.
Mid-morning	Mixed raw vegetable platter with lemon juice.
Lunch	Jacket potato (eat jacket) with ham and 1 green pepper; grapes and 1 pear.
Supper	Grated carrot and apple salad; grilled cod steak with 1 tbs brown rice; 1 orange.

Day 2
Breakfast	Half a grapefruit; 1 boiled egg; bread from allowance.
Mid-morning	2 dried figs.
Lunch	Brown rice and tomato salad (mix 2 tbs cooked brown rice with 2 sliced tomatoes, chopped onion, basil or thyme, vinegar and a little oil, and chill).
Supper	Small steak or hamburger with mushroom, cucumber and apple salad; 1 pear.

Day 3

Breakfast Orange juice; small helping bran cereal with sliced apple on top; bread from allowance.

Mid-morning 2 tomatoes.

Lunch Shredded white cabbage, carrot and apple salad mixed with yogurt and vinegar; 1 hard-boiled egg.

Supper Small grilled lamb chop with fresh spinach or broccoli and grilled tomatoes; stewed apple with crunchy oatmeal or bran topping.

Day 4

Breakfast Grilled tomatoes on toast from allowance topped with grated cheese and bran.

Mid-morning Raw celery and carrot sticks.

Lunch Small portion drained tuna tossed with chopped cucumber, green pepper and apple in lemon juice.

Supper Chicken leg baked with coating of wholemeal breadcrumbs, a dash of curry powder and seasoning; one carton natural yogurt liquidized with 75g cucumber to make a sauce; green salad.

Day 5

Breakfast Grapefruit with cinnamon topping; 1 scrambled egg topped with wheatgerm on bread from allowance.

Mid-morning Fresh fruit salad.

Lunch Salad of chopped beetroot and onion, cooked butter beans and French beans, all tossed in vinegar with seasoning; 1 apple.

Supper Slimmer's tomato soup with wholemeal bread croutons; small portion chilli con carne; green salad with lemon juice dressing.

Day 6

Breakfast Orange juice; muesli and 1 tbs bran with milk from allowance.

Mid-morning Bread from allowance with cucumber or tomato.

Lunch Slice of lean ham; a salad of mixed raw vegetables (carrots, cucumber, cauliflower, etc.).

Supper Herring cooked in oatmeal; green beans or broccoli; 1 apple.

Day 7

Breakfast Fresh fruit salad with yogurt and nuts; bread from allowance.

Mid-morning Hard-boiled egg, bread from allowance.

Lunch 1 bowl calorie-reduced minestrone with bran sprinkled on top; salad of chicory and tomato with walnuts.

Supper Roast turkey or chicken with cabbage, broccoli or spinach; carrots; boiled potato (leave skin on).

The vitamin C diet

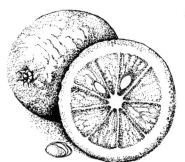

Here's a diet that's specially suitable for vitamin C shy men. It's designed to trim your tum in two weeks and get you in the mood to enjoy fresh, summer foods. It cuts down alcohol, but realistically allows half a bottle of wine a day or a couple of shorts or pints. So it's quite easy to fit into your life, even if you're a high-powered chap with clients to entertain or a heavy manual worker who just has to wind down at the pub after work or at lunchtime! The diet contains plenty of vitamin C and minerals to fill you full of bounce and some tasty salad recipe ideas to tempt men who are notoriously anti-salads.

For lunch, I suggest sandwiches – but you can reverse the evening meal with the lunches if you're having a business meeting. Do try if possible to arrange meetings within office hours during the fortnight – you'll get more work done before your holiday if you nibble a sandwich at your desk. No one – not even *you* – needs two big cooked meals a day. Sorry!

Follow the diet for two weeks. Before or with each meal drink a glass of diluted lemon juice with water, mineral water or soda to help educate your naughty, carbohydrate-obsessed palate away from sweet, starchy, *fattening* foods. You won't like it one bit at first but it will grow on you, I promise.

Daily allowances Unlimited water or lemon juice (such as PLJ) in water, low-calorie drinks, tea or coffee without sugar. Your milk allowance is half a pint and it should be *skimmed*. You are allowed half a bottle of dry wine (red or white) *or* 2 pints of bitter *or* 3 shorts (pub measures!) with low-calorie mixers only. Don't cheat. You may eat two pieces of fresh fruit from the following list: apple, orange, pear, peach, large grapefruit, 100g raspberries or strawberries.

Breakfasts Have one of these every morning:
• Boiled egg and crispbread with low-fat spread and yeast extract.
• Half grapefruit, two rashers streaky bacon, grilled, with grilled tomatoes.
• 25g any breakfast cereal plus 100ml skimmed milk (additional to allowance).

Lunches Choose one sandwich only and add unlimited salad nibbles (tomato, lettuce, etc.); use two slices wholemeal bread, and do *not* spread the bread with butter.
• Cheese and pickled onion: mix together 35g grated Edam cheese, 1 level tbs Slender Mayonnaise (see page 61) and one chopped pickled onion.
• Salmon with olives: flake 65g canned salmon with 2 stuffed olives, chopped and 1 level tsp low-calorie seafood sauce. Spread on bread and top with tomato slices before covering with the other slice.
• Curd cheese with gherkins: chop 3 small gherkins and mix with 65g

curd or cottage cheese. Spread bread with yeast extract before making up sandwich.

- Chicken and mango chutney: chop 50g cooked chicken, mix with 1 slightly rounded tbs mango chutney and 1 tbs chopped cucumber.
- Prawn and tomato chutney: mix together 65g peeled prawns, 1 slightly rounded tbs tomato chutney and 1 tbs chopped cucumber.

Suppers You *must* choose a salad at least three nights a week.

Hot Meals

- 150g cod, haddock or plaice, grilled.
- 1 trout, brushed with 1 tsp oil and grilled.
- 100g liver, grilled or casseroled in stock.
- 2 lambs' kidneys and 2 rashers streaky bacon, grilled.
- 1 large chicken joint, grilled.
- 100g ham steak with drained pineapple ring.
- 100g lean pork fillet, casseroled.
- 100g beef, casseroled.
- 100g chicken livers simmered in stock with tomato purée and mushrooms.

To any of the above add unlimited broccoli, brussels sprouts, cabbage, cauliflower, celery, onions, leeks, tomatoes, runner beans, French beans or courgettes, and 1 small jacket or boiled potato or two tablespoons rice. Do *not* add butter to the vegetables, just steam or boil them very lightly.

Salads

- Coleslaw and cheese: shred 65g white cabbage and mix with 25g carrot and 50g Edam cheese, both grated. Add 2 tbs natural yogurt and 1 tbs Slender Mayonnaise and season to taste.
- Chicken, orange and cucumber: cut 75g cooked chicken into half-inch pieces; peel and chop 1 medium orange and 50g cucumber. Mix together 1 tsp chopped mint, 2 tbs natural yogurt, 1 tsp lemon juice and seasoning. Combine the chicken, orange and cucumber into the dressing.·
- Curried egg and prawn: shell and chop 1 large hard-boiled egg. Peel and dice a one-inch section of cucumber. Mix together 3 level tbs natural yogurt, 1 tsp lemon juice, $\frac{1}{4}$ level tsp curry powder, a few drops Tabasco, salt and pepper. Toss egg, prawns and cucumber in the curry dressing.
- Corned beef and vegetables: cook 100g frozen mixed vegetables according to packet instructions, drain and cool. Dice 65g corned beef and mix with vegetables and 1 tbs Slender Mayonnaise plus 1 tsp lemon juice and seasoning.

Add to any of the above unlimited salad greens – lettuce, chinese cabbage, chicory, watercress, cucumber – or tomatoes, and lemon-juice dressing.

Note If you're entertaining, any of the above salads will go down a treat with weight-conscious guests. Just add French bread and boiled new potatoes for the non-dieters. But *no* nibbling!

The high protein diet

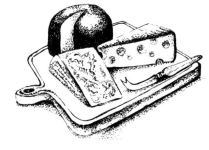

This is suitable for healthy, pregnant mums and anyone who wants to feel good, but *not* lose weight. It includes all the goodies that you need if you feel below par. Most of us don't realize that the body needs a re-charge of essential vitamins and minerals when it's under stress, and stress can mean anything from coping with the demands of a growing baby to bearing up after your partner walks out.

The diet has an approximate daily calorie total of 1700 with ample quantities of vitamins A and D. There is a daily pinta as well as calcium-rich cheese (mums-to-be who can't stand milk should step up their cheese intake to ensure strong teeth and bones in the baby). This diet would be equally suitable for any male in a sedentary job who wants to shed a few pounds, but it's a little short on carbohydrate for he-men in tough manual jobs.

Daily allowances 1 pint milk; 1 digestive biscuit (nibble it when you wake up if you're pregnant!). Cut spirits out altogether but allow yourself the occasional glass of wine or, better still, stout – a good source of vitamin B and iron.

Day 1

Breakfast 50g grated Edam cheese and 1 sliced tomato grilled on 1 slice wholemeal bread; 1 apple.

Lunch Tomato Cocktail (see page 57); 2 slices corned beef; 75g sweetcorn; 1 fruit yogurt.

Supper Paprika Goulash (see page 60); 1 tbs boiled rice; 1 tbs cottage cheese with a dry biscuit.

Day 2

Breakfast Small bowl bran cereal topped with sliced banana and milk from allowance; 1 slice wholemeal bread spread with yeast extract.

Lunch Half grapefruit; 1 slice wholemeal bread topped with 2 tbs cottage cheese and 1 sliced tomato; watercress and cucumber salad.

Supper Grilled lean pork chop; 1 baked potato; boiled spinach or broccoli; 1 natural yogurt.

Day 3

Breakfast 1 rasher back bacon grilled with 1 tomato and 25g mushrooms; 1 slice wholemeal bread with a scraping of butter.

Lunch 100g tuna fish; large mixed salad; 25g Cheddar cheese with 1 dry biscuit.

Supper 100g grilled liver or kidney with mushrooms; 50g each carrots and cabbage; 1 fruit yogurt.

Day 4

Breakfast   Tomato Cocktail; 1 boiled egg; 1 slice wholemeal bread and scraping of butter.

Lunch   1 bowl of calorie-reduced tomato soup topped with 50g grated Edam; 1 slice wholemeal bread; 1 orange.

Supper   Small grilled herring; 1 slice wholemeal bread and scraping of butter; 1 fruit yogurt.

Day 5

Breakfast   Small bowl bran cereal topped with a sliced pear and milk from allowance; 1 slice wholemeal toast with a scraping of butter and honey.

Lunch   2 slices of ham rolled round 50g cottage cheese and 50g chopped pineapple and served on lettuce; orange, date and mint fruit salad.

Supper   Haddock Bake (see page 59); grilled tomatoes; baked apple stuffed with raisins.

Day 6

Breakfast   2 eggs scrambled with milk from allowance and a little butter on 1 slice wholemeal toast and topped with grated cheese and 1 sliced tomato.

Lunch   1 cubed apple, 50g cubed Cheddar and 1 chopped carrot tossed in natural yogurt and lemon juice and piled on lettuce; 1 slice wholemeal bread and a scraping of butter.

Supper   Tomato Cocktail; 100g Mexican Casserole (see page 60); 100g green beans or broccoli; 1 orange.

Day 7

Breakfast   1 thin slice melon; small bowl muesli with milk from allowance.

Lunch   Tomato Cocktail; 100g roast chicken; mixed salad; small baked potato; 25g Cheddar cheese with 1 dry biscuit.

Supper   1 poached egg on 1 slice wholemeal toast; tomato salad; 1 fruit yogurt.

The fruit and veg diet

This month-long diet is based on fresh, low-calorie seasonal fruits and vegetables, plus some lean meat and fish. It's rich in things to help make you feel good as well as look good – including vitamin A (in carrots, apricots, eggs, green vegetables) which will help prepare your skin for a safe suntan. You'll notice that it is relatively *low* in fats (especially animal fats) and there may be rather less meat than you are used to.

    How much weight will you lose? Unfortunately, it's impossible to say how much an individual will lose on any given diet. If you're an active type, expect to lose around 1.82kg in the first week, then about .91kg a week afterwards. Fluid loss accounts for the dramatic reduction over the

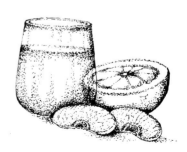

first week. Of course, if you normally eat huge meals three times a day, you may lose much more.

Dry wine is allowed on the diet, which should help beat the alcohol bug that often ruins dieting efforts. But, quite frankly, you won't stay the course if you try to combine the diet with too many parties. There is a limit to how much temptation the human psyche can stand! Try to be really busy during the week, and spend the weekends doing something *active*; sports, walking, swimming. Never miss a meal or save up two meals for the evening – you're bound to come unstuck. If possible, get your nearest and dearest to join you in the diet. If they won't co-operate, at least serve up *your* meals at night for them – with the addition of fattening extras like bread, potatoes, and pasta which you should put on their plates only, *not* in a communal serving dish which you may be tempted to dig into.

Daily allowances Half a pint low-fat, skimmed milk for use in tea or coffee; 12g butter for spreading on bread; half a bottle dry wine (red or white) which you may wish to save up for special occasions!

Breakfasts Choose one every day. You can drink tea or coffee with milk from allowance (use an artificial sweetener such as Hermesetas or Sweetex if you must – but do try to give up sugar completely!).
● Soak 50g dried apricots in 100ml strong black tea overnight. Add artificial sweetener if needed and serve with 1 tbs muesli.
● Scoop out the flesh of half a grapefruit and mix with 75g cottage cheese, seasoning and 1 grilled diced rasher of bacon; pile back into grapefruit skin and serve with 1 crispbread and butter from allowance.
● 2 chipolatas, 2 tomatoes and 4 mushrooms dotted with butter from allowance and grilled.
● 1 carton natural yogurt; 1 egg, boiled; 1 slice wholemeal toast with butter from allowance.
● 1 small banana, 1 apple and 25g Edam cheese.
● Orange juice; 1 scrambled egg (butter from allowance) on 1 slice wholemeal bread.
● Cottage Cheese with Melon (see page 58); 1 slice wholemeal bread and butter from allowance.
● Grapefruit juice; Piperade (see page 58).

Lunches Drink tea or coffee with milk from allowance or a glass or two of your wine allowance, and choose from the following:
● Salmon Avocado (see page 57); 1 orange.
● 2 slices corned beef; grated carrot and lettuce salad; 1 fruit yogurt.
● Melon Picnic (see page 58); a few grapes.
● Greek Cheese Salad (see page 61); 1 banana.
● Mushroom omelette (2 eggs); mixed salad (no mayonnaise).
● Small portion any grilled fish; green salad with lemon-juice dressing.

- 1 bowl low-calorie soup; open sandwich of one slice lean ham on 1 slice wholemeal bread (butter from allowance) topped with tomato slices.

These lunches are packable (with the exception of the omelette and fish), so use your slimming month as a time for picnics in the park during the lunch break *or* for working extra hard! If you have a lunch date, choose fish or an omelette with salad. Never, ever miss out on lunch.

Suppers Choose one every day, and use the rest of your wine allowance:
- Scrambled Avocado (see page 58); 1 slice wholemeal toast with butter from allowance.
- Avocado Stuffed Peppers (see page 57); tomato and onion salad with lemon juice and garlic dressing; 1 banana.
- Chicken leg roasted with fennel, onion and chicken stock; 50g each green beans and carrots; 1 apple.
- Cauliflower cheese, using 50g Edam in a sauce made with milk from allowance and 25g flour; 3 grilled tomatoes; fresh fruit compôte.
- Yogurt Stroganoff (see page 60); orange and date salad.
- 4 slices any white meat; a large mixed salad with Slender Mayonnaise (see page 61); 1 orange.
- Ginger Kidney Casserole (see page 60); cucumber salad; 1 fruit yogurt.
- Cod steak cooked in foil with mushrooms, lemon juice, herbs and seasoning; 1 baked potato; a green salad.
- 2 slices lean ham or beef with Courgette Salad (see page 61).
- 25g hard cheese with 1 crispbread and butter from allowance.

Note Choose the simplest meals (e.g. cold meat, cauliflower cheese) when you're rushed for time, but do try to plan ahead at least twice a week – choosing the kidney recipe or the Yogurt Stroganoff (see recipes on page 60), for instance, which can be dressed up if you have guests. At weekends it's fine to swap them for lunches if you wish to entertain at lunchtime. Remember that salads *can* be large without detracting from the effectiveness of your diet ... so *don't* stint the lettuce, green peppers, celery and cucumber in your diet. Go easy on salt, though – it does make you retain fluid, and herbs or lemon juice can be just as tasty without the 'puffy' effect of a high salt intake.

Three-day diets

It's unwise and unnecessary to go on a very drastic diet for longer than three or four days, but there are times when a short semi-fast can be good for you. For instance, when you've been on a round of business lunches or supper parties and feel that you're bulging all over, or when you simply must lose a few pounds for a very special occasion.

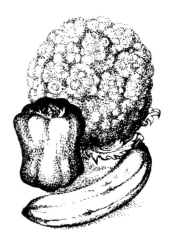

If you decide to follow one of the diets below, do be sure that it's during a period when you won't be required to do much physical or mental work – a long weekend is a good idea. Arm yourself with a gripping book and don't glue yourself to the television – the ads will make you rush to the larder. Relax and enjoy yourself. You'll find that your body feels delicious and your brain reaches a kind of 'high' after a couple of days.

You can mix the diets if you like, by using the fruit juice diet on Day 1, the soup diet on Day 2, and so on.

Daily allowances You may drink unlimited water and diet soft drinks on all three diets.

The Fruit Juice Diet
Breakfast   1 glass mixed (unsweetened) vegetable juice.
Mid-morning   1 large glass orange juice; 1 carton natural yogurt.
Lunch   Tomato juice cocktail made with 1 carton natural yogurt, 1 large glass tomato juice, lemon juice and Worcestershire sauce blended and served with ice and sprigs of mint.
Mid-afternoon Mixed orange and grapefruit juices; 1 slice wholemeal bread.
Supper   Grated carrots mixed with shredded cabbage and tossed in lemon juice with a few nuts and raisins; 1 large glass mixed vegetable juice.

The Soup Diet
Breakfast   1 bowl calorie-reduced soup, any flavour, with 1 slice wholemeal bread.
Mid-morning   1 bowl chilled slimmers' tomato soup; 1 cube hard cheese.
Lunch   1 bowl calorie-reduced soup; 1 small tin baked beans.
Mid-afternoon 1 glass mineral water.
Supper   1 bowl of calorie-reduced soup; 1 bowl fresh fruit salad.

The Raw Vegetable Diet
Breakfast   2 sliced tomatoes and 1 tbs cottage cheese on 1 slice wholemeal bread; black coffee or lemon tea.
Mid-morning   Unlimited scrubbed carrots, celery and cucumber.
Lunch   A large salad of raw mixed vegetables tossed with 1 tbs cottage cheese and lemon juice.
Mid-afternoon Unlimited scrubbed raw vegetables.
Supper   100g grilled white fish and a mixed salad with lemon-juice dressing.

Recipes for sociable slimmers

This selection of recipes is linked to the diets in this book, but they are all suitable for inclusion in any calorie-controlled slimming plan. They are low in calories and easy to prepare – perfect for lunch or dinner parties when you want to have a delicious meal in smart surroundings *without* ruining your diet. You can easily give them to non-slimming guests without feeling that you are depriving them of anything – in fact, the dishes are so scrumptious that they'll never know they are eating a low-calorie meal.

Tomato Cocktail

(Serves 4) 1 425g tin Italian tomatoes; 1 stick celery; 2 tsp lemon juice; 1 tsp each chopped parsley and Worcestershire sauce; salt and pepper.

Put all the ingredients into the blender for 30 seconds, then strain into a saucepan and simmer for five minutes. Adjust seasoning, chill and serve in individual glasses garnished with lemon.

20 CALORIES PER GLASS.

Italian Vegetable Soup

(Serves 4) 1 large onion; 1 small turnip; 2 carrots; 1 green pepper; 1 leek; 2 bouillon cubes; 800ml water; 50g alphabet pasta; 2 tbs chopped parsley; 50g grated Parmesan cheese; salt and pepper.

Make up stock with cubes and boiling water, combine with chopped onion, turnip, carrots and green pepper and simmer for 20 minutes. Add the chopped leek and simmer for a further 10 minutes. Finally add the pasta and simmer until tender. Sprinkle with parsley and Parmesan and serve.

200 CALORIES PER BOWL.

Salmon Avocado

(Serves 1) half avocado; 1 tbs Slender Mayonnaise (see page 61); $\frac{1}{2}$ tbs natural yogurt; $\frac{1}{2}$ tbs tomato ketchup; 90g tinned salmon; cucumber slices and watercress, sprigs.

Mix mayonnaise, yogurt, ketchup and flaked fish thoroughly. Pile into avocado cavity and garnish with cucumber and watercress.

445 CALORIES PER PERSON.

Avocado Stuffed Pepper

(Serves 1) half avocado; 100g cottage cheese; 1 red or green pepper; lemon juice; salt and pepper; lettuce.

Blend the cheese and avocado flesh, stir in lemon juice and seasoning. Cut top off pepper, de-seed and fill with mixture. Chill for at least an hour, and serve with lettuce.

300 CALORIES PER PERSON.

Scrambled Avocado

(Serves 1) half avocado; 1 tomato; 1 rasher bacon; 2 eggs; 1 dsp chopped parsley; salt and pepper.

Skin and chop tomato. Chop bacon and fry in its own fat until crisp; add the beaten eggs and tomato and stir until mixture thickens. Season and pile into avocado cavity.

450 CALORIES PER PERSON.

Cottage Cheese with Melon

(Serves 1) half a small melon; 175g cottage cheese; cucumber slices; chives or ground ginger for flavouring; salt and pepper.

Season cottage cheese and pile into melon cavity. Chop chives or sprinkle ginger over the cheese and garnish with cucumber slices. Chill before serving.

200 CALORIES PER PERSON.

Melon Picnic

(Serves 1) half a melon; 100g cooked and chopped chicken; 1 green pepper; 3 tbs Slender Mayonnaise (see page 61); 1 tbs chopped mint; paprika, salt and pepper.

Remove the flesh of the melon with a teaspoon, discarding the pips; de-seed green pepper and slice thinly. Mix both with mayonnaise, season and replace in melon skin. Garnish with mint leaves and paprika, and wrap in cling film for travelling.

270 CALORIES PER PERSON.

Piperade

(Serves 4) 75g low-fat spread (e.g. Outline); 1 large onion; 1 green pepper; 1 red pepper; 4 tomatoes; 4 eggs; 1 tbs vegetable oil; 1 tsp thyme; salt and pepper; 4 slices starch-reduced bread.

Melt two-thirds of the low-fat spread in a frying-pan. Add the chopped onion, peppers and tomatoes, thyme and seasoning. Cover and cook gently for ten minutes or until soft. Make 4 hollows with the back of a spoon in the mixture and break 1 egg into each; cover and cook gently until set. In another frying-pan melt the rest of the low-fat spread and vegetable oil. Cut bread slices into triangles and fry until golden. Serve each person with a quarter of the piperade topped with an egg and garnished with fried bread.

265 CALORIES PER PERSON

Cheese and Broccoli Flan

(Serves 6) 150g shortcrust pastry; 150g Edam cheese; 200g lightly boiled broccoli, chopped and drained; 1 onion; 1 large or 2 small eggs; 125ml milk; 50g butter; pinch of nutmeg; salt and pepper.

Roll out the pastry and line an eight-inch flan dish; bake blind in a fairly hot oven (200°C, Gas Mark 6) for fifteen minutes, then reduce heat to 175°C or Gas Mark 5 for ten minutes. Chop onion and cook gently in the butter. Beat the egg, and mix with the milk, broccoli, nutmeg, seasoning and onion. Take out the cooked flan case, place half the sliced Edam over the bottom, spoon over the broccoli mixture and cover with the remaining cheese. Bake for 20 minutes or until cheese is brown and the flan is set.
354 CALORIES PER PERSON

Baked Fish with Pasta
(Serves 4) 500g filleted white fish; 1 small tin tomatoes; 2 glasses dry white wine; 200g pasta shells; juice and grated rind of half a lemon; 25g grated Edam cheese; 1 tbs chopped parsley; salt and pepper.

Arrange fish in an oven-proof dish, season, pour on wine and add chopped tomatoes; cover with greaseproof paper and bake in a moderate oven (175°C, Gas Mark 5) for 20 minutes. Cook pasta shells until tender, drain and toss in lemon juice and rind, parsley and seasoning. Arrange round fish, sprinkle with cheese and melt in oven or under grill.
200 CALORIES PER PERSON

Haddock Bake
(Serves 4) 225g smoked haddock fillet; 175g cooked sweetcorn; 25g flour; 150ml low-fat reconstituted milk; 150ml water; 25g butter; 175g grated Edam cheese; 1 tsp each mustard powder and lemon juice; salt and pepper; parsley sprigs and lemon segments.

Poach fish for 7–10 minutes, then drain and flake, reserving water. Make a white sauce with the butter, flour, fish water and milk. When smooth and thick stir in fish, sweetcorn, cheese, mustard powder, lemon juice and seasoning to taste. Pour mixture into ovenproof dish and grill until golden. Garnish with lemon segments and parsley.
320 CALORIES PER PERSON

Chicken Lasagne
(Serves 4) 75g lasagne; 150g chopped cooked chicken; 1 tin calorie-reduced chicken soup; pinch of nutmeg; 50g toasted breadcrumbs; 1 tsp lemon juice; 25g butter; salt and pepper.

Cook lasagne in plenty of boiling water until tender; drain and refresh in cold water, drain again. Heat soup, chopped chicken, nutmeg, lemon juice and seasoning. Grease a six-inch square dish and line with a layer of lasagne. Put a layer of the chicken mixture on top, then another of lasagne, another of chicken and another of lasagne. Top with remaining sauce, sprinkle with breadcrumbs and melted butter and bake in a hot oven (200°C, Gas Mark 6) for half an hour.
300 CALORIES PER PERSON

Paprika Goulash

(Serves 4) 450g lean shin of beef or braising steak; seasoned flour; 1 tbs vegetable oil; 1 onion; 1 green pepper; 2 tbs tomato purée; pinch each of nutmeg and mixed herbs; 1 clove garlic; 2 tbs paprika.

Cube meat and toss in seasoned flour; fry in a non-stick pan. Crush garlic, chop onion and pepper and add to pan with flavourings. Cover and simmer for about 1½ hours or until meat is tender (you may have to add a little stock or water if the pan becomes dry).

305 CALORIES PER PERSON

Yogurt Stroganoff

(Serves 4) 500g rump steak; 2 onions; 200g mushrooms; 1 tbs vegetable oil; 1 425g tin Italian tomatoes; 1 tsp each Worcestershire sauce and French mustard; 1 carton natural yogurt; 3 tbs chopped parsley.

Cut beef into thin strips, onions into rings and mushrooms into slices. Heat oil in a non-stick pan and fry beef briskly. Add onions and mushrooms and fry gently until soft. Add tomatoes and flavourings and cook gently for 15 minutes or until beef is tender. Stir yogurt into mixture, garnish with parsley and serve.

340 CALORIES PER PERSON

Mexican Casserole

(Serves 4) 500g lean stewing steak; 1 large onion; 1 carrot; 1 tbs vegetable oil; 1 small can Italian tomatoes; 1 small can baked beans; 275ml stock; 1 tbs Worcestershire sauce; pinch chilli powder; bouquet garni; salt and pepper.

Cube meat and place in casserole. Fry chopped onion and carrot gently in oil then add to casserole with tomatoes, stock and flavourings. Cook in moderate oven (175°C, Gas Mark 5) for 1½ hours. Add baked beans and cook for further 15 minutes.

340 CALORIES PER PERSON

Ginger Kidney Casserole

(Serves 4) 450g ox kidney; 50g low-fat spread; 275ml calorie-reduced ginger ale; ½ tsp ground ginger; 1 tbs vinegar; 1 beef stock cube; 1 tbs diet blackcurrant jam; 1 tbs cornflour; 2 tbs water; salt and pepper.

Remove hard core of kidney and cut into small pieces. Melt the low-fat spread in a large saucepan, fry the kidney gently until sealed. Add ginger ale, flavourings, vinegar and stock cube and bring to the boil, stirring constantly. Simmer for 40 minutes or until kidney is tender, then stir in jam and let it melt. Mix the cornflour with the water, add to the pan and bring back to the boil, stirring all the time. Cook for 2 minutes, adjust seasoning and serve.

200 CALORIES PER PERSON

Courgette Salad

(Serves 4) 450g courgettes; 40g low-fat spread; 1 clove garlic; 1 onion; 2 large tomatoes; 1 tbs vinegar; 1 tbs vegetable oil; salt and pepper.

Dice courgettes and blanch in boiling water. Melt the fat in a frying-pan, add garlic and onion and cook gently until soft. Add the courgettes, season and cook for 5 minutes then cool. Peel and de-seed the tomatoes and chop the flesh. Mix oil and vinegar together and combine with courgettes and tomatoes. Serve cold.

90 CALORIES PER PERSON

Greek Cheese Salad

(Serves 4) 1 lettuce; 12 black olives; 100g fetta or 175g cottage cheese; 2 tomatoes; 1 slice white bread; 25g low-fat spread; 1 tbs lemon juice; salt and pepper.

Tear lettuce leaves into small pieces. Halve and stone olives. Crumble the fetta. Peel the tomatoes and chop the flesh, removing the seeds. Trim crust off bread, dice and fry in low-fat spread until crisp. Put lettuce into a salad bowl or individual dishes and pile the other ingredients on top.

100 CALORIES PER PERSON

Pasta and Chicken Salad

(Serves 4) 100g pasta shells or other shape; 100g chopped cooked chicken; 1 red pepper; 2 stalks celery; 1 lettuce; 1 tbs vegetable oil; 2 tbs lemon juice; 1 tbs chopped parsley; pinch of nutmeg; salt and pepper.

Cook pasta until tender, drain, and while still hot add oil and lemon juice and toss. Leave to cool. De-seed and slice pepper, slice celery and onion and add to pasta with chicken and seasoning. Arrange lettuce leaves in a salad bowl and pile mixture on top.

250 CALORIES PER PERSON

Tomato Sauce for pasta and plain boiled vegetables

(Serves 2) 1 425g can Italian tomatoes; 1 onion; 1 clove garlic; juice of half a lemon; 1 tbs chopped parsley; 1 tbs vegetable oil; salt and pepper.

Chop onion finely and cook gently in oil until soft. Add remaining ingredients and cook for 15 minutes, mashing tomatoes with a fork. (Make this sauce in double or treble quantities before you start the Pasta Diet and deep freeze until needed.)

42 CALORIES PER HELPING

Slender Mayonnaise

(Serves 2) 1 carton natural yogurt; 1 tbs calorie-reduced mayonnaise; 1 tbs lemon juice; 1 tsp French mustard.

Blend or whisk all ingredients until smooth. You can make this in double or treble quantities if you are entertaining.

30 CALORIES PER HELPING

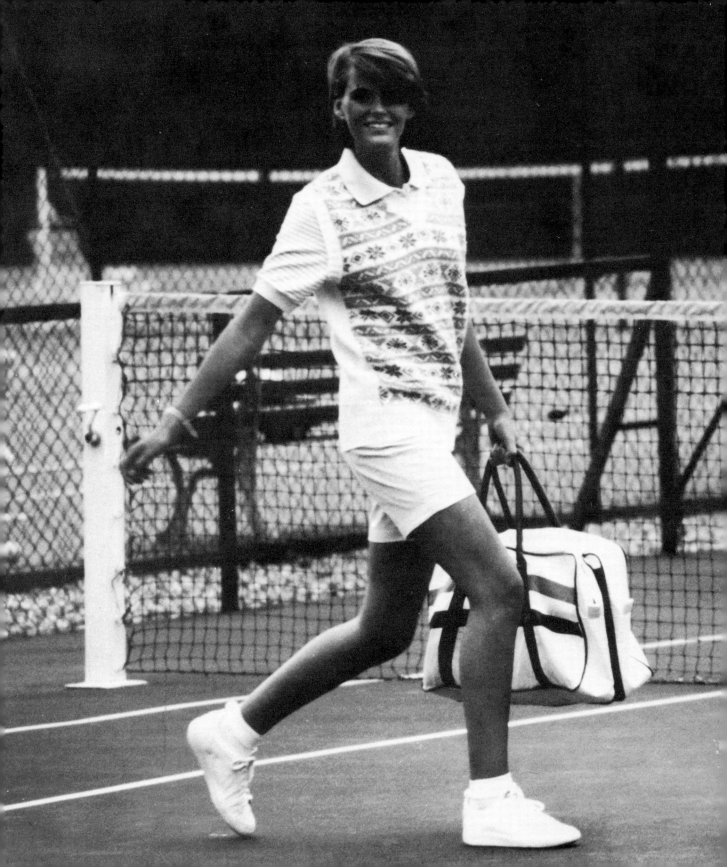

4 Get Glowing

If you want to slim fast – get *glowing*. Your body must work hard to burn off excess calories and to rev up the metabolic processes which help you slim; you can make it work that little bit harder by going jogging, walking, running on the spot, breathing correctly and by discovering the luxury of *massage*. All these methods are good ways to stimulate circulation and make sure that oxygen and nutrients carried in the blood stream reach all parts of your body. They also help warm up your body for more intensive forms of exercise.

Don't believe that deep breathing and luxurious massage can help you slim? Well, *breathing* is actually a form of exercise; if you take deep breaths you exercise your rib cage, midriff, diaphragm and the invisible corset of muscles which hold your tummy in. Deep breathing also gives a valuable boost of oxygen to the brain, making you feel brilliant, alive and less in need of the added stimulus of *food*. Massage may be highly relaxing, but it is also a sensational way of whipping up circulation and encouraging you to be *aware* of your body, bulges and all!

During your slimming stint, and afterwards, you should try to step up all these methods of body stimulation. Use them as a warm-up before more intensive forms of movement (it is very important to avoid starting a strenuous exercise programme when your muscles are cold). Run up and down stairs a few times, for instance, before doing a workout; jog around the block before whizzing off to a hard squash session; walk through the park to your dance class or yoga lesson.

Massage won't *remove* fat, but it will help revitalize sluggish circulation and give your metabolism a useful 'jolt' to encourage weight-loss. It will also help you relax (important if tension and stress are contributing to your eating problems) and give you a sensual, pampered feeling which will help you become more aware of your body, and even to *like* it a little more! If you can, try a professional massage once in a while.

One form of massage, aromatherapy (which involves the use of essential oils from plants and pressure at certain vital parts of the body) has been used very successfully to treat such problems as poor circulation, bad skin, constipation and cellulite. The last problem is one which is, at last, being recognized as a form of obesity which differs from other fat problems; in cellulite, the fat forms on hips, thighs and upper arms and gives a characteristic 'orange peel' appearance to the skin. Many cases have been treated with a combination of intensive aromatherapy massage, low-salt diet, and rigorous exercise. If *you* have this kind of stubborn fat, then it's well worth trying the massage techniques explained in this book and, if possible, investing in a course of

Boost your circulation with movement. Exercise in the park at lunchtime!

aromatherapy massage sessions (see addresses on page 111).

I am going to take you through two massage treatments; one with a partner, the other alone. Yes, it really is possible to give yourself a massage, although it isn't as thorough as the kind that can be obtained with a partner to do the hard work! It's useful, however, when it just isn't possible to share the experience.

Try either technique once or twice a week while you are trying to lose weight, to encourage fat mobilization and increase body awareness. Once you've slimmed down, you should still find time for a weekly massage. Just before you go on holiday, step up the massage sessions again to two or three a week, using body oils to soften your skin and prepare it to face the sun. You'll find that tanning is easier, and your skin feels far less dry and sore after swimming.

Top to toe massage

You need a partner, a *warm* room, a bed or padded table with a towel on top for your subject to lie on, and oils. Try to use a vegetable oil such as olive, safflower or soya bean oil, and add a few drops of scented essence to give a delicious fragrance. These essences can now be bought at many health and beauty shops, and make fabulous perfumes as well as a delicious additive for massage. They can also have a dramatic effect on the subject; try these brews to help specific problems:

To tone muscles and relieve aches mix ten parts juniper oil, with five parts each lavender oil and rosemary oil.
To relax your subject completely mix ten parts geranium with five parts lavender and four parts marjoram oils.
To make your subject lively and amorous mix seven parts bergamot, seven parts sandalwood and three parts each of rose and jasmine oils. Beware – this has a very powerful aphrodisiac effect!

Make sure your hands are clean, fingernails well filed, and palms dry. If your hands are cold, it's friendlier to warm them up before starting the massage. Have plenty of tissues at hand to mop up any oily residue after the massage, although this will be less than you think; the oils will soak into the skin pretty rapidly. Make sure your oil is blended properly and is in a non-spill container. Right, ready? Now get your subject to strip off completely and lie on his back on the towel.

Massage technique Keep your hands relaxed throughout the massage, and use your *whole body* to apply pressure, otherwise, you'll end up feeling exhausted, with very tired arms indeed. Mould your hands as you work to fit the contours of your subject's body, and maintain an even, rhythmic pressure. This will come with practice. Never pour the oil directly on to his body; pour it on to your hand, and then rub it in. Don't talk too much while you work; massage should be a relaxing experience, a form of communication through *touch* not words.

1 Start by holding your palms lightly against his forehead, for a second or two, then begin massaging it with the balls of your *thumbs* in circular movements. Don't press too hard.

2 Now, very gently, lift his head slightly and turn it slowly to the left. Rotate the heel of your right hand against the top of his shoulder and . . .

3 Stroke it up towards the back of his neck. Then turn his head to the right, and concentrate on the left shoulder.

4 Spread a little more oil over his chest, tummy and sides of his body. Now stand behind his head and place both hands firmly on the middle of his chest, fingers pointing towards his feet. Glide both hands forward, pressing firmly on the chest, more lightly on the tummy, then separate hands and bring them back along the sides of his torso. Repeat ten to fifteen times.

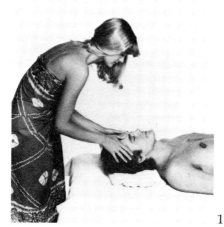

1

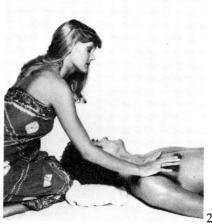

2

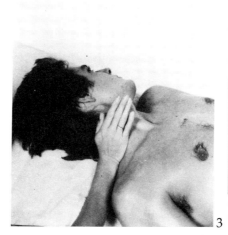

3

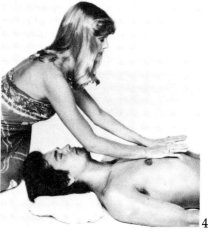

4

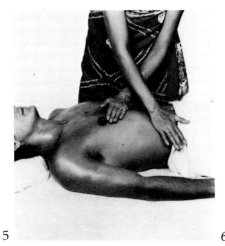

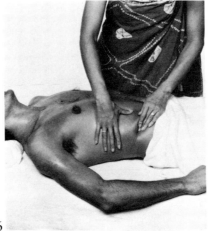

5 Move to his side and make slow circular movements with the palm of your left hand, moving clockwise. Now follow up with the palm of your right hand and keep it going for about six to twelve full circles.

6 Now reach across to the side of his body opposite you and grasp (gently, please!) as much loose flesh as you can between the thumb and fingers of one hand. Pull it up towards you, slowly letting it slip from your fingers and following up with the other hand in a 'kneading' movement. Keep it up for twenty double strokes, then walk around to the other side and repeat.

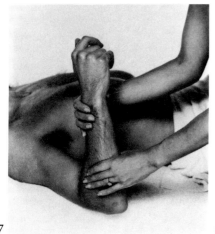

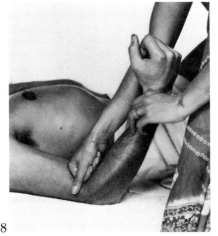

7 Raise his forearm, elbow still on the bed and make a ring around his wrist with your thumb and forefinger. Now glide your hands gently down to his elbow, release the pressure and bring hands back to his wrist again; repeat five times.

8 Now very gently rub your knuckles against the inside of his elbow.

9 Place his hand against your shoulder, raise his arm off the bed and repeat the first stroke from elbow to shoulder level, finishing with knuckle massage under his armpit. Repeat the whole sequence with the other arm. This process is called 'draining' and it really does help to relieve tired arms and increase circulation. Wonderful for anyone who wields a spade, typewriter or pen for a living!

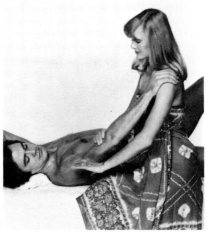

10 Move to face his *feet*, and place both hands round one ankle. Now glide them up the leg to the top, leaning over to exert pressure and increasing that pressure over the thigh area. Now pull your hands right down to the ankle again. Repeat with the other leg.

11 Lift one leg gently so the knee is bent, foot flat on the bed, and rub the underside of the thigh with your forearm, left to right all the way up, right to left all the way down. Now vigorously rub and pinch the whole thigh area. Repeat with the other thigh.

12 Get him to turn over on to his tummy (you may have to wake him up first!). Now make a rapid criss-cross movement, using both hands, all the way up and down the back of one leg. Stiffen your fingers a little to make a claw shape and work briskly over the top of the thigh and buttock area, concentrating on any fatty bits. Finish the leg with softer, soothing strokes, then repeat the whole process on the other leg.

13 Spread more oil on his shoulders, back and sides, come round to the top of his head and concentrate on his shoulders and back. Place your hands on his shoulders, fingers lightly touching his spine, wrists outwards. Make strong strokes down his back to waist-level, pull hands back up his sides and repeat ten times.

14 Knead the muscles curving from his neck to his shoulders between your thumbs and forefingers (both hands at once). This movement can be a bit painful, so be firm but gentle.

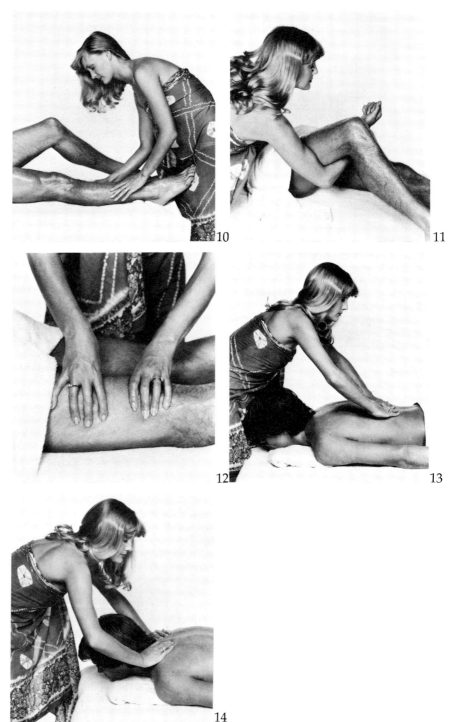

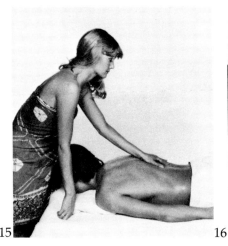

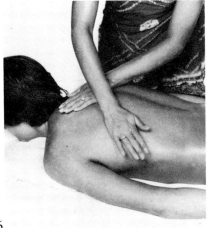

15 Trace his spine, using your forefinger and thumb either side of the spine itself, from shoulders to the very base of the spine; repeat five times.

16 Now come round to one side, place both hands on the further shoulder and make big circular movements, ten or even twenty; then repeat on the other side.

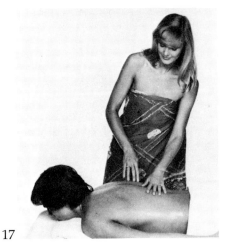

17 Finish the massage, using both hands at once to trace a series of very light, fingertip strokes right down his body, neck to feet.

If your subject is asleep, just cover him lightly with a towel and leave him to rest.

If he has to get up immediately, rub his body very gently with a tissue to absorb any excess oil before he dresses. If possible, get him to wear something casual and loose so he can allow the complete feeling of relaxation to flow over his body without restrictions. Don't worry, he won't be so relaxed that he's unable to work properly! Within half an hour or so, he'll feel the true benefits of increased circulation, and his brain will be bursting with oxygen and brilliance!

Go-it-alone massage

For this relaxing treatment for one you need privacy (use a bathroom or bedroom and lock the door); a towel to lie on; body oil; tissues; a warm dressing-gown to slip on afterwards.

1 Start by lying down on your back on the floor or bed. Now massage your temples and forehead with your fingertips in circular movements. Let your ring fingers touch very lightly on these points (one after the other): outer corners of the eyes, inside the bridge of the nose, on cheek-bones, at the points where the jaw meets the ear-lobes.

2 Still lying down, press your fingertips either side of the top of your spine, working down as far as you can reach, then back up again.

3 Now sit up, and let your head hang forward as you make tiny circles below the base of your skull with your fingertips. Let one shoulder and arm go limp, then reach across and behind your head with the other hand. Press your fingertips really hard across the top of the shoulder blade. Repeat with the other shoulder and hand.

4 Now lie down again, and spread some oil over your tummy. Rub it in with your palm in a circular, clockwise movement. Then knead and squeeze flab and spare flesh on your tummy and midriff using the fingers and thumb of both hands. Make dragging movements with both hands, working across your body from your midriff down to your hips. About twenty or thirty strong movements (your tummy may be rumbling by this time!).

5 Bring one knee up to your tummy and knead and rub your foot with both hands, working plenty of oil between the toes and using your knuckles to rub the soles and arches fairly firmly. This is great for tired feet, and helps to keep your feet smooth and corn-free. Repeat with the other foot.

6 Sit up and knead and slap your thighs. Lean forward bending your knee slightly and grasp your ankle with both hands, stroke your leg in long sweeping movements, right up to the upper thigh. Repeat five times, then switch to the other leg.

7 Now roll over on to your tummy, and pinch and knead your bottom for a few seconds – be really firm. Slap it till it tingles. Bottoms often get sluggish and grey looking as well as bulgy; this is a good movement to use if you intend to bare all on the beach in summer.

8 Lie still, facing downwards, for a few minutes to recover, then stand up and slap your whole body very lightly, from the top of your head to your toes. You'll feel relaxed, invigorated, glowing. Wipe off any excess oil, and try to relax for a half-hour or so before dressing.

Note Some of the movements, especially the kneading ones, can be performed in the bath. They aren't quite so painful underwater, and really do help to get rid of flab.

Boosting your circulation

Exercise and muscle-toning machines can be a valuable help in keeping you trim, but they are no substitute for the real thing! Some are good for *monitoring* your progress (such as the cycling machines which include pulse and energy-testing meters) and letting you see just how fit or unfit you really are. Here's a guide to the machines available, and what they can do for you:

Cycling and rowing machines are good for testing stamina and endurance and exercising legs and tummy muscles, and arms in the case of rowing machines. Doctors recommend their use for heart patients who want to build up their stamina gradually. Some machines also include a cardio-tester, which can register the pulse and indicate the amount of energy used for pedalling. Prices start at about £100.

Faradic muscle toning machines are used in hospitals for restoring muscle tone to damaged limbs, and in the home and at health farms to tone up sluggish muscles. The basic machine consists of eight body pads which are strapped into position over the appropriate muscles. The machine is turned on, and you feel a faint tingling sensation which intensifies as the power increases. This may feel unpleasant at first, but most people soon get used to it. However, you do need skill to place the pads over the correct area; a bad operator can stretch the skin. Personally, I'm not keen on women using these too soon after having a baby; skin is slack after being stretched and vulnerable to this kind of strong contracting action. The disadvantage with these machines is that once you stop using them, you will quickly become flabby once again. Prices start at £150.

Jogging machines are designed for those who like to walk or jog, but hate going outside in the rain. You get the same exercise using one of these machines which consist, basically, of two rollers and a strip of canvas. The rollers are electrically-driven and adjustable for slow or fast joggers. Muscles exercised include abdominals, bottom, thighs, arms. However, there is the disadvantage that the view is rather restricted! Prices start at about £240.

Massage machines range from the large belted vibrating machine right down to the very small electric massagers with a variety of attachments. The large machines used at health clubs are not really suitable for home use; they simply help you feel tingly, and whip up circulation. They will *not* 'whittle away' your waistline or bulgy bottom, unless you combine the treatment with diet and exercise. The same thing applies to smaller vibratory massagers, though these can be beneficial in dealing with cellulite, which clings to hips, thighs and arms. A daily massage plus a sensible diet with lots of water to drink, fresh vegetables, fruits and a *minimum* of fatty foods, tea, coffee, and sugary foods, can really help move this type of fat. Experts suggest you use a special anti-cellulite cream or gel containing extract of ivy with the machine *or* manual massage with a special rubber-headed plastic massager, but to have an effect massage needs to be both intense and regular. After the bath is a good time. Cost: about £17 for a hand vibratory massage machine, and rather less for one of the hand-massaging kits.

Jacuzzis, whirlpools and saunas are deliciously pampering devices. You may think that a jacuzzi is way out of your price-range, but there are now a number of firms making bath attachments which whip up a wonderful whirling, jacuzzi-type effect in your own bath. You feel tingly and stimulated, and circulation is given a valuable boost. While this effect does not slim you down, you can use it after exercising to prolong the metabolic 'revving-up' which physical effort promotes.

The dry heat of a sauna is good for cleansing your body, and (yet again!) stimulating circulation. It's also relaxing, and some people find that the perspiration lost during a sauna gives them a morale-boosting weight-loss. However, you must remember that this is purely temporary; once fluid is replaced, your weight will go right back to normal again. Doctors are concerned that too many overweight, out-of-condition fatties leap into saunas without considering the shock that such intense heat gives to the system. Remember, don't stay in too long, don't take a sauna after a meal, don't take a sauna at all if you feel droopy, have a history of heart trouble or have been drinking. Cost: about £300 for a jacuzzi-type bath attachment, and over £1,000 for a home sauna cabinet.

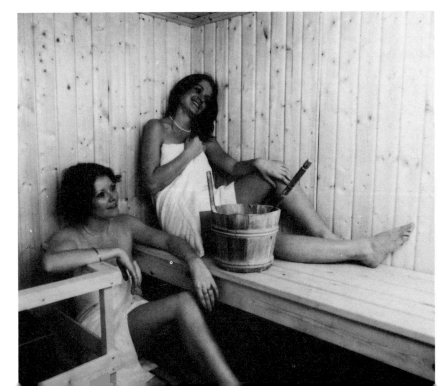

A sauna is a good deep-cleansing treatment, but don't stay in too long.

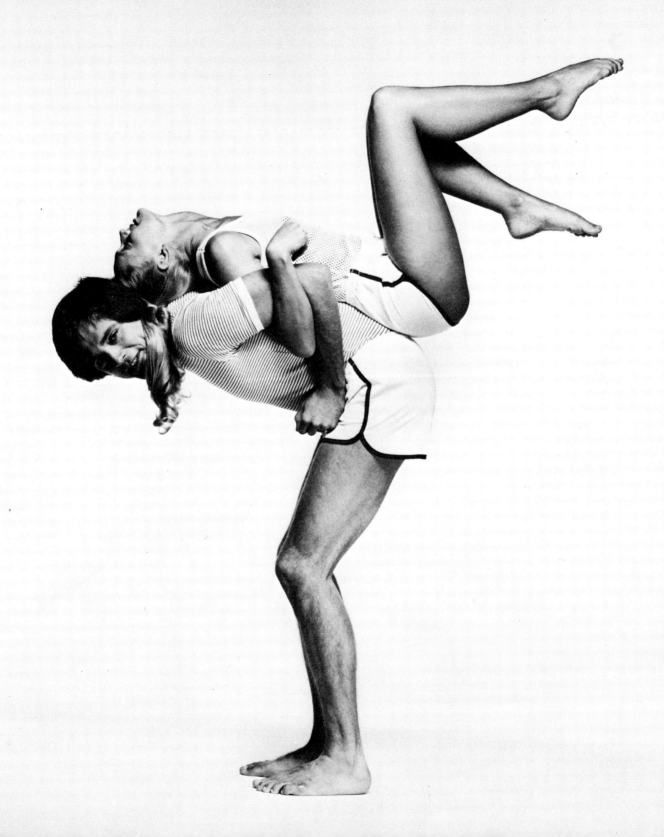

5 Exercising

Depressed by the very sound of the word exercise? Don't just sit there, *do* something! Try to think of exercise as *fun*, as a positive pleasure in life, not a chore. It really is possible to incorporate a fair amount of exercise into your life without too much trouble and the rewards are *tremendous*. Not only will you feel the positive benefits in your shape, your vitality, your energy – but you'll also feel mentally refreshed after every single exercise session, whether it's a yoga workout at lunchtime, a swim in the pool, or just a rapid walk around the block with the dog.

Each exercise routine in this section of the book is designed to stimulate your *interest* as well as make you feel energetic. They have been selected because they are effective, easy and don't need any special equipment or instruction.

Slimming through exercise

Over *half* the human body is composed of muscle fibres, and improving their condition is an important part of any slimming programme. Muscles pull your mouth upwards in a smile, make your fingers move to pick up a cup of coffee, your legs move to run for the bus. They are made of three different kinds of tissue: cardiac tissue (found in the heart, the most important muscle in the body), smooth muscle tissue which lines the walls of the intestines and arteries, and striped muscle tissue which forms the skeletal muscles like those of the arms and legs. If you looked at striped muscle tissue under a microscope, you'd see lots of tiny cylindrical fibres, bound by connective tissue and encased in a fibrous sheath.

Muscles are also divided into two groups: involuntary and voluntary. The *involuntary* muscles get on with the job without conscious messages from us; the intestine muscles take care of food once it has been eaten, the arterial wall muscles pump blood from the heart and the heart itself just goes on quietly beating without any conscious message from the brain. But the *voluntary* muscles need stimulus from the nervous system before they can contract, and set a movement in motion. In other words, your brain has to direct operations! Even when you do something as simple as laughing, your brain must direct the appropriate muscles to tweak the corners of your mouth upwards. Directed any muscles to move about lately? I bet it's ages since you directed your buttock muscles to do *anything* other than lie in a squashy mound on that chair!

What happens after the direction is given? The muscles are attached to the skeletal bones by short, tough tendons. Once the message is received, the muscles contract pulling the appropriate part of the skeletal frame

Togetherness is finding a friend to share your exercise campaign!

with them. The tendons prevent them from coming adrift, and the frame itself moves smoothly with the help of the joints between the bones – hips, shoulders, elbows, knees, etc.

Muscles should be kept in a constant state of partial readiness for this effort, ready for the full contraction which comes with that message from the brain. If your muscles are in this happy state – you have good muscle 'tone'. 'Tension' is simply a state where the muscles are contracted more than the limit required for perfect tone, leading to problems like backache, headaches, shoulder-ache. Very slack muscle tone (sounds like yours?) usually means that extra exertion is difficult or painful and, most important for slimmers, it can also lead to pockets of *fat* being formed around the slack muscle. This is why exercise can be so beneficial for your body; it not only tones up those slack muscles but positively *discourages* those pockets of fat from forming. There is also evidence that the metabolic 'revving up' processes which are triggered off by exercise go on being effective for some considerable time after the exercise is ended. This is why the rather discouraging figures produced about the calorie-burning effects of exercise (e.g. you'd have to walk to Brighton to burn off one pound of body fat!) are not strictly correct. Exercise is much *more* effective in a get-slim campaign than many people realize.

The major muscle groups
Sternomastoid These are each side of the neck. They act independently to bend the head sideways and turn the head and they act together to bend the head on to the chest.
Exercise by head bending and rotation.
Trapezius This is a triangular-shaped muscle across the back of the neck and shoulders which draws the shoulders together and downwards and acts as a brace for the shoulders. Bad tone can aggravate 'dowager's hump' and rounded shoulders. The trapezius takes a heck of a lot of strain if you, like me, sit for long hours hunched over a hot typewriter.
Exercise by shoulder circling, backward arm swings.
Deltoids These stretch over the top of the shoulders, covering the shoulder joints like epaulettes. They raise the arms up to shoulder level sideways and, in conjunction with other muscles, help rotate the arms and raise them to the front and back.
Exercise by any arm-raising movement or weight-lifting, and sports like gymnastics, climbing, tennis or boxing.
Latissimus dorsi This is a broad muscle which stretches across the back into the back of the arms. It helps to draw the arms down and back and to rotate them. It also pulls the trunk up towards static arms (e.g. rope-climbing).
Exercise by pulling arms down and backwards, preferably against some kind of resistance, and sports like rowing, climbing.
Brachialis These stretch across the front of the upper arms, across the

joints. They help to flex the arms in conjunction with the biceps. Exercise by arm-bending against resistance such as weight-lifting; digging and shovelling earth are good too.

Biceps At the front of the upper arms, these are well-known even to anti-exercisers! They turn the hands palm upwards to bend the arms. Exercise by using the same routine as you do when working the Brachialis muscles.

Triceps At the back of the upper arms, these straighten the elbows. Exercise by pushing arms against resistance and by throwing, pushing, punching, and sports like cricket, baseball, javelin-throwing, boxing.

Wrist flexors On the fronts of the forearms, these help bend the palms of the hands towards you. Exercise by hand gripping, pushing wrists forwards. Sport like golf, tennis, bowls, squash, badminton.

Wrist extensors On the backs of your forearms, these pull the back of the hand away from you. Exercise by wrist clenching, gripping and handstands (if you're energetic enough!).

Pectorals These are in the upper chest, above the breast. They help to draw the arms across the body and rotate the arms inwards. They help support the breasts and should be exercised regularly to prevent the droops. Exercise by strong resistance of the hands against an immovable object (such as pushing against a typewriter or wall), rotating arms inwards and pushing inwards (pushing hands together in front of your chest, for instance).

Serratus anterior At the sides of the upper rib-cage, these muscles help you push with your arms. Exercise by pushing against resistance, or by activities like mowing the lawn, carpet-sweeping or vacuum cleaning.

Intercostals Between the ribs in two distinct layers, these help you breathe by raising and lowering the ribs as you inhale and exhale. Exercise by deep and regular breathing.

Abdominals This group includes the internal and external obliques and transversalis, and forms a muscular 'corset' three layers thick between the diaphragm and the pelvis. They bend the trunk from side to side, rotate it, and support the stomach. If they are strong, your tum is flat and firm. Exercise by bending and twisting the trunk, leg raising and 'sit-up' exercises, dancing, gymnastics and sports involving throwing.

Rectus Abdominis These extend down the middle of the abdominals to the pubic bone and they bend the trunk forwards. Exercise by bending forward, sit-ups, leg raises, sports involving forward movements such as rowing.

Erector spinae These extend each side of the whole length of the spinal column. They help the spine to move smoothly and keep the trunk erect. Exercise by back-arching, raising the trunk from a forward position.

Buttock group This group of muscles extend all over the seat. They pull the thighs sideways and backwards, revolve the legs and some of them help raise the trunk from a stooping position.

Exercise by raising legs backwards and by contraction (try it: contract buttocks hard, hold for a count of ten then relax. This is one of the most effective anti-bulge exercises for your bottom because it can be done absolutely *anywhere*. Aim for a hundred clenches a day if you have the spreads, and see the difference!).

Hamstring group These are at the rear of the thighs. They bend the knees and help rotate them outwards and extend the legs backwards. They are vulnerable because walking and sitting don't exercise them enough and sudden strain can cause damage.

Exercise by toe-touching, leg stretching.

Quadriceps femoris At the front of the thighs, these extend the knees and bend the hips.

Exercise by leg straightening and kicking movements such as football, rugby and activities like running, walking, climbing.

Tibialis anterior At the front of the lower legs, these raise toes and feet up and towards you and turn the feet inwards.

Exercise by foot bending and circling, and turning feet up and inwards.

Calves group At the back of the lower legs, the calves group raise your heels, and point the toes downwards.

Exercise by heel raising, toe-pointing, standing on tip-toes, walking, running, jumping, dancing.

Adductors These are on the insides of the thighs and are used to pull upper legs *inwards*. Because these are not used too often, fat often accumulates around them.

Exercise by making love, riding, swimming (not all at once!).

Abductors On the outside of the thighs, these muscles insert into the soft tissues of the lower thigh and have no bony connection. Fat is very easily accumulated on them. They are used to carry the leg outwards and rotate it inwards.

Exercise by walking and running, always keeping the feet pointing for-wards. If you've noticed a fatty accumulation on the outside thighs, make a real effort to walk with feet forwards (most people tend to walk with toes outwards, Charlie Chaplin fashion) and you'll find that thighs become trimmer.

Bath exercises

Not *quite* ready for the rigours of that daily dozen? Ease yourself into the exercising habit painlessly with a bathtime exercise routine. It's effective, and far less demanding than any other kind of keep-fit session because the buoyancy of the water supports your body weight rather like a cushion. That's why hydrotherapy is used in hospitals for patients who need the gentlest-possible muscular therapy.

Make sure your bathroom is warm, but keep the water at a comfortable temperature; if it's too hot, you could feel faint or sick. Be sure to do the exercises on an empty tummy. The bathwater level should be just up to your neck when you lie back in the bath. A bath pillow is a good idea for some of the movements.

1 This is a good exercise for strengthening tummy, thighs and lower back muscles.

Lie back in the bath, arms by your sides, feet together, head resting comfortably on the bath pillow. Now slowly raise your arms to the horizontal position, bending your knees and lifting your feet at the same time. Point toes, hold the position for a count of six, then lower feet and arms slowly. Repeat ten times.

2 This one tightens tummy muscles, strengthens legs, hips, back, shoulders and arms.

Lie back in the bath, legs stretched out and toes wedged under the taps, hands by your sides.

Sit up slowly and stretch your arms to try and touch your toes, leaning forward so your face comes down towards the water. Hold for a count of ten, then lie back slowly. Repeat ten times.

3 This is super for tummy muscles, less painful than the usual abdominal exercises.

Lie back again, feet resting on the bottom of the bath, knees bent, hands floating by your sides. Now pull in your tummy muscles, almost as though you were trying to touch your spine with your navel. Hold for a count of three, then release. Repeat five times, resting between each exercise. Breathing is important here: breathe out deeply before you pull in your tummy muscles, breathe in again as you release them.

4 This is a really effective thigh-tightener.

Lie back in the bath, hands resting on the bottom. Draw your right heel back along the bottom of the bath towards your bottom. Straighten the leg, bringing up your left heel at the same time. Keep the movement going rhythmically, ten with each leg, then ten with both legs together.

5 If you want to trim your waistline, try this exercise in the bath every day for a week, measuring your waist at the beginning and end of the week. You could lose up to one inch.

Sit up in the bath, resting your feet on the bottom, legs slightly apart. Clasp your hands behind your head, making sure your back is straight and head held high. Twist your trunk slowly to the right, going as far as is comfortably possible. Hold for a count of three, then return to starting position and relax for a further count of three. Repeat, twisting to the left this time. Repeat whole movement ten times.

6 Here's a final bath exercise, this time for your hips.

Lie back in the bath, resting on your forearms and elbows at the sides of your body. Slide back your feet so they are flat on the bottom of the bath. Slowly raise your hips and bottom (easier than it sounds, because of the buoyancy of the water), and swing your hips gently and evenly from side to side. Ten swings!

Stretchercises

These exercises are good for hunched, tired bodies, kept cramped in a sitting-down position all day. They literally 'stretch' your limbs, helping you recover from occupational hazards such as rounded shoulders from slaving over a desk or bench all day, or flabby tum from humping small children on your hip. Recommended for late afternoon, when your body feels it needs a brisk trot through the park but you are surrounded by problems designed to keep you indoors!

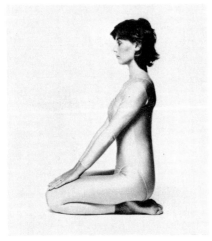
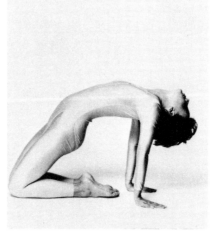
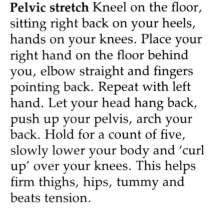

Pelvic stretch Kneel on the floor, sitting right back on your heels, hands on your knees. Place your right hand on the floor behind you, elbow straight and fingers pointing back. Repeat with left hand. Let your head hang back, push up your pelvis, arch your back. Hold for a count of five, slowly lower your body and 'curl up' over your knees. This helps firm thighs, hips, tummy and beats tension.

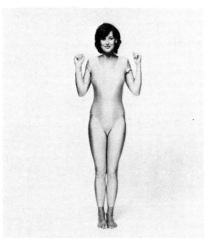
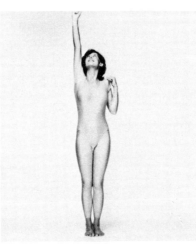

Arm stretch Stand with feet slightly apart. Now, bend your elbows and bring your hands up to shoulder height, hands curled into loose fists. Thrust first one arm rapidly then the other upwards with a flinging movement, keeping fist curled. Do a total of ten times. This helps keep arms flexible (so it's good for tension caused by typing, or writing, or even brick-laying), and gets rid of pent-up tension. Do it when you feel like hitting someone!

Total stretch Lie on the floor, feet slightly apart, arms out at an angle of 90° to your body. Now point your toes and push your legs downwards, one at a time, then reach out to the side, first with your left hand, then with your right. Relax for a few seconds, then bring your hands by your sides, palms down. Pushing down on your forearms, raise your chest off the floor, arching your back. At the same time, pull your head under until you are resting on the very top of it. Now shift your weight until most of it is being carried by your buttocks. Hold until you begin to feel twitchy (about one minute) breathing normally. Relax slowly. This does wonders for neck and upper back tension, helps circulation, stimulates the thyroid.

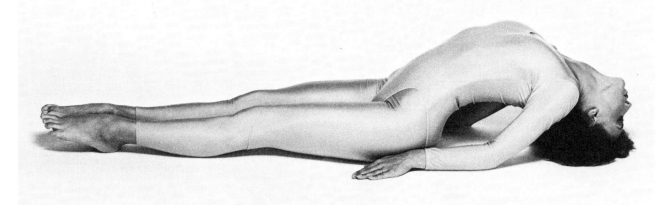

Leg stretch Sit on the floor, legs outstretched and as far apart as possible without straining or falling over. Keeping knees flat, back straight, place your hands on one leg. Slowly slide your hands down towards your feet, bending forward from your waist, tummy well in. When you've reached a point that's comfortable, let your head hang down, clasp your legs and raise your elbows. Hold for a count of five, then relax. Helps constipation, menstrual pain, firms thighs and makes spine more flexible.

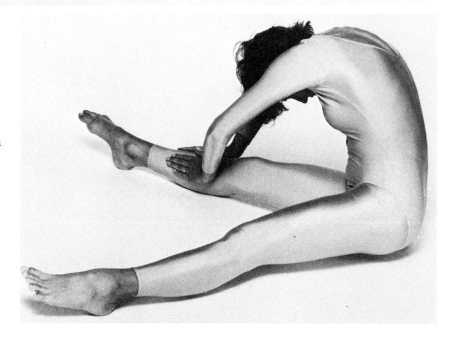

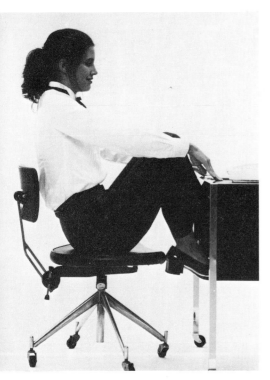

Try exercising in your office. It'll help beat backache – and make you slim.

Isometrics

Wherever you go, whatever you do, you can do isometrics. The principle is simple: the muscle is contracted through pushing, pressing, pulling or squeezing against an immovable object. This contraction helps to strengthen the muscle – and has the advantage of being easily combined with other physical activities. They are a favourite with people who are unable to exercise in a highly energetic way. Using this technique, you can extend your exercise programme to include some useful, effective isometrics that can be done *outside* the home – in the office, in the bus queue or in your car.

This is an exercise method which should appeal to people who swear they simply have not got the time to devote to a regular programme: if you practise these movements often enough you find that they become almost automatic. And they take up no time for you – do them while doing something else, answering the telephone, for example. Some of the exercises included in the programme have the added advantage of relaxing and toning tired muscles. So you will find that you feel less fatigued and irritable at the end of a working day.

These isometric exercises have been deliberately chosen so that they can be done unobtrusively, at your office desk or during a car journey. Be sensible in your approach – fit the exercises in as and when they seem appropriate. There is no need to stop working while you do them, but remember that while the movements themselves may be unobtrusive you will reveal your secret if you allow the effort to show on your face. Clenched teeth or rolling eyes will not make the exercise either easier or more effective.

• To strengthen pectoral muscles.
Sit at your desk (or a table, about five feet wide) with back straight, feet together. Spread your arms and grip the outside edges of your desk. Squeeze in hard with your hands. Hold for a count of six, then relax. Take a deep breath before starting to squeeze hands, then breathe out slowly as you hold the position. Rest, then repeat five times.
• To strengthen inside thigh muscles.
Sitting comfortably on a straight-backed chair with arms relaxed, grip a waste-paper basket between the inner edges of your feet. Squeeze feet together as hard as you can. Hold for a count of six, then relax. Breathe regularly throughout the exercise. Repeat five times.
• To strengthen flabby upper arm muscles.
Sitting at your desk with back straight and feet together, place the palms of your hands flat on the desk-top about one inch apart. Press down as hard as you can, almost as though you were trying to force the table into the floor. Hold for a count of six, then relax.

Now place the palms of your hands beneath the edge of the desk. Keep your elbows tucked in against your sides and press upwards as hard as you can (if the table is light, weigh it down with a heavy typewriter). Hold for a count of six, then relax. Breathe in as you start to press your hands up or down, out as you hold the position. Repeat the whole exercise five times.

- To strengthen arm, shoulder and back muscles.

While taking a telephone call, stand an arm's length from a convenient wall. Hold the receiver to your ear with one hand and push the palm of the other hand hard against the wall. Hold for a count of six, then relax. Breathe regularly throughout the exercise (you will be talking, too). Repeat five times, then change hands and repeat a further five times.

- To strengthen upper arm, shoulder and back muscles.

Stand with your back to a tall filing cabinet (or wall), about nine inches away from it. Keeping legs straight, feet slightly apart and arms straight reach backwards and press the palms of your hands flat against the filing cabinet. Now push back hard with both hands. Hold for a count of six, then relax. Breathe in as you start to push, out as you hold the position. Repeat five times.

- To strengthen the upper leg rear muscles.

Stand straight with your back about one foot from a filing cabinet. Raise your right foot until it rests under the handle of the second to bottom drawer of the filing cabinet. Rest your left hand on a chair back for balance. Now press your right heel hard against the drawer handle pulling up against it. You should feel the back thigh muscles contracting. Hold for a count of six then relax. Breathe regularly throughout the exercise. Repeat five times.

- To strengthen upper back and stomach muscles.

Sit comfortably on a straight-backed chair, feet together, back straight. Now part your knees and place your feet firmly on the floor about one inch apart. Place the palms of your hands flat on your thighs. Keeping arms straight, press downwards strongly pulling in your stomach muscles at the same time. Hold for a count of six, then relax. Breathe in as you start to press down, and hold your breath as you count six. Breathe out as you relax. Repeat five times.

- To strengthen wrists and forearms.

Stand near a bus-stop or any vertical post and grip the post with both hands, right hand above the left, and arms bent. Now move your arms as if to twist the right hand in an anti-clockwise direction and the left hand in a clockwise direction, but resisting the effort as you do so. Hold for a count of six then relax. Breathe regularly throughout the exercise. Repeat five times.

- To strengthen arm and pectoral muscles.

While waiting in a traffic jam, use the time for some simple exercises. Grip the steering wheel at the nine o'clock and three o'clock positions, and squeeze in your hands hard. Hold for as long as possible, then relax. Breathe regularly throughout the exercise. Repeat as often as time allows.

- To strengthen back muscles.

Still sitting in that traffic jam, grip the steering wheel in the position just described. Now straighten your arms and push back as hard as possible against the seat behind you. Hold for as long as possible, then relax. Breathe regularly throughout the exercise. Repeat as often as time allows.

- To strengthen thigh muscles.

Holding the steering wheel in the same position as for the last two exercises, press your heels back hard against the front of the seat. Hold for as long as possible, then relax. Breathe regularly throughout the exercise. Repeat as long as the hold-up allows!

Yoga asanas

Yoga is one of my favourite forms of exercise because it is gentle, non-strenuous and improves your breathing and reduces tension as well as helping you get in shape. Yoga asanas aren't really exercises at all, they are postures; slow, controlled movements are necessary to obtain each posture, and it's the *quality* of the posture that's all-important, not the number of repetitions or the speed at which you perform.

All good yoga teachers stress the importance of finding your own level; never straining, simply trying to follow the instructions carefully and performing to the best of your ability without undue effort. It's essential to join a class if you're going to take up yoga seriously, but in the meantime here is a complete yoga programme of ten exercises. Practise each one carefully, on the floor or on a practise mat. Try each asana once on the first session, then twice on your second session, working up to about five repetitions. Make sure you haven't eaten anything for at least one and a half hours before the session. Wear a leotard and tights or loose T-shirt and shorts. No shoes, please!

The corpse This is the posture of deep relaxation. Adopt it for a few minutes at the beginning and end of the session. It's a useful posture for times when you need to relax and replenish your strength; try it after a busy day at work when you have a tiring evening ahead, or at midday when you have a hectic afternoon in front of you. When you feel frazzled and irritable, try the corpse for a few minutes.

1 Lie on your back, feet apart, head well back.

2 Place your hands on the floor, palms up, away from your body, and let your feet flop open.

3 Close your eyes, and try to imagine your body sinking into the floor. Hold the position for a count of one hundred (longer if you have time), then get up very slowly. Your whole body will feel refreshed and revitalized.

The complete breath This helps your lungs function efficiently, and recharges your body with a marvellous boost of oxygen to your brain – use it when you want to be brainy or inspired!

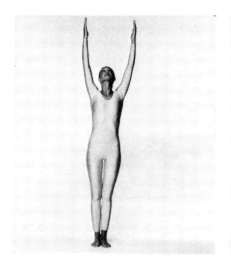 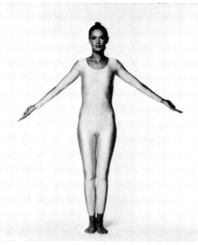

1 Stand with your back straight, feet together, head erect, hands hanging down loosely at thigh level.
2 Inhale deeply, bringing your hands up slowly, palms uppermost, letting your tummy expand and looking up, until your palms touch above your head.
3 Now exhale slowly, lowering your arms back to your sides and *pushing* the air out through your mouth as you pull in your tummy. This takes practice at first.

The cobra This classic, graceful asana helps your spine remain flexible, relieves tension in your shoulders, tightens tummy and buttock muscles, improves posture – and makes you feel *wonderful*.

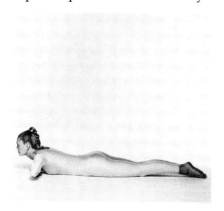 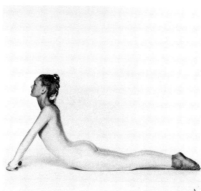

1 Lie on the floor on your tummy, quite relaxed, hands by your sides, head on one side. Close your eyes and relax for a moment.
2 Slowly, bring your hands round so they are tucked in by your chest, fingers pointing inwards.
3 Lift your head up very slowly, letting your hips rest on the ground, your back curve gently. Look upwards and push down on your hands, straightening your arms. Hold the position for a few seconds, then lower your body gently to position 2.

The coil This increases strength and mobility in your neck and spine, firms and trims your bottom and helps flatten your tummy.

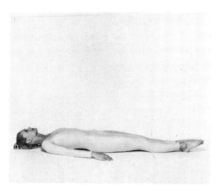
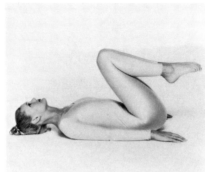

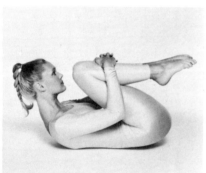
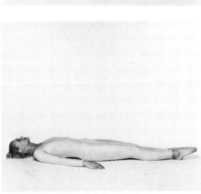

1 Lie flat on your back, legs and feet together, arms by your sides, palms down.
2 Bend your knees, raise your feet off the floor, toes pointed, and bring them in towards your chest.
3 Lock your fingers, loop your hands over your knees and pull them towards you, raising your head and shoulders off the ground.
4 Hold the position for a count of five, then lower your head to the floor and relax for a few seconds before unlooping your arms and bringing your legs and arms back to position 1.

The locust This is a superb asana for wobbly bottoms and upper thighs,
but it is quite difficult, so do relax completely afterwards.

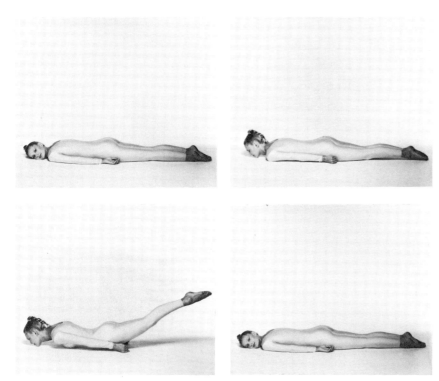

1 Lie on your tummy, hands by your sides, palms upwards, head on one side so your cheek rests on the floor. Let your heels drop open, bend your elbows slightly and *relax*.

2 Bring your legs and feet together, place your chin on the floor and straighten your arms, making your hands into fists.

3 Take a deep breath, push down hard with your fists and raise your legs, keeping your knees straight and your feet together. Raise them as far as is comfortable (it won't be very far at first), hold the position for a count of five, then lower them very slowly.

4 Relax before repeating the exercise.

The bow This is a good bust-firming asana, which also strengthens the arms, shoulders and neck, and helps beat midriff bulge.

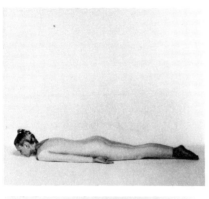

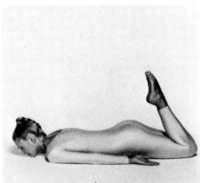

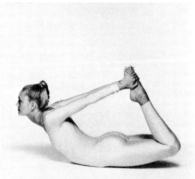

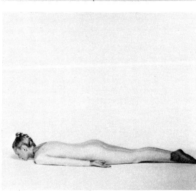

1 Lie flat on your tummy, chin on the floor, arms by your sides (palms up), feet together, toes pointed.

2 Bend your knees, bringing your feet in as close to your body as you can.

3 Now reach back with your hands and grab your toes. Keeping your elbows straight, pull your feet and raise your head. Then, gently but firmly, push your feet back towards the floor, pulling your body up and back. Look up to the ceiling and count five.

4 Let your chest sink slowly down, keeping hold of your feet. Release your feet, and lower them slowly to the floor. Relax completely for a few seconds.

The squat This is good for balance and posture, and slims and firms your legs. It also helps cure knee and ankle stiffness and is an ideal exercise after a day's shopping or a night's disco-dancing.

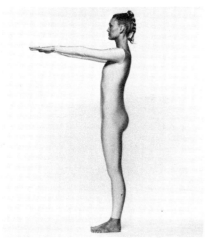 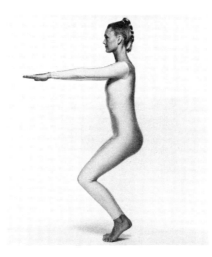

1 Stand with back straight, head up, feet together, arms by your sides. Raise your arms to shoulder level, palms down.
2 Keeping your back straight, rise up on to the balls of your feet, bending your knees at the same time. Go down right on to your heels (no wobbling!).
3 Hold the position briefly, then straighten up very slowly, finally lowering your heels and dropping your arms by your sides.

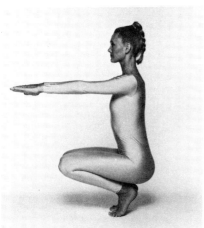

The camel This eases shoulder strain, makes your back more supple, and tones and strengthens the front thighs.

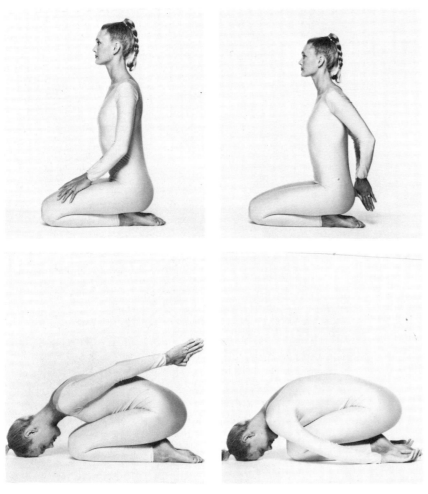

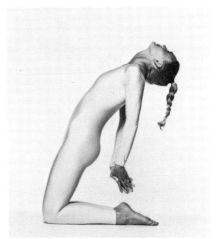

1 Sit back on your heels, holding your thighs lightly, elbows bent, back perfectly straight.
2 Very slowly, place your hands behind you with fingers pointing backwards.
3 Push up your chest, tummy and bottom, making your body into a curved shape, and lifting your bottom off your feet.
4 Slowly arch back on to your heels as in position 1, then let your body bend forward, so your forehead touches the floor in front of you.
5 Now let your arms rest limply. Hold this comfortable position, breathing quietly, for a few seconds before straightening up.

The plough This is a wonderful back-stretching exercise, but it *must* be done slowly and carefully.

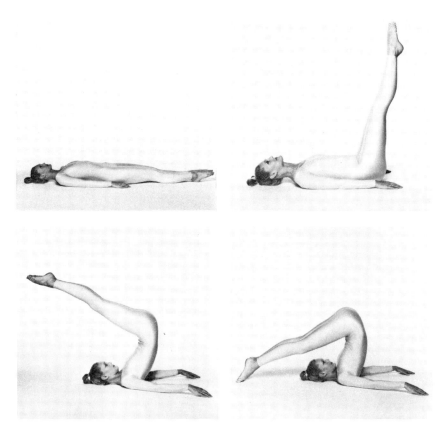

1 Lie flat on your back, feet together, toes pointed, hands by your sides, palms downwards.
2 Raise your legs, keeping your knees straight, feet together, and pushing down on the floor with your hands to give leverage.
3 Very slowly, push your legs over as far as they will go (don't try to touch the floor at first, no need to rush it). Count five.
4 When you can touch the floor, hold that position for a count of five, then slowly roll down, bringing your legs smoothly down to the floor. Relax completely in the corpse position.

Note When you can do this exercise easily you can extend it by bending your knees after position 4 to touch the floor each side of your head. Hold for a count of five then roll down as before.

Two's company!

Here are six exercises to try with a willing partner. They're fun, easy and good for you. Try them on the beach or in the garden in summer, in the bedroom in winter. Encourage each other to stay the course:

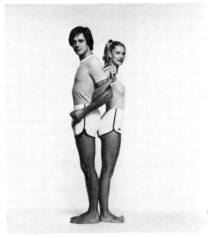

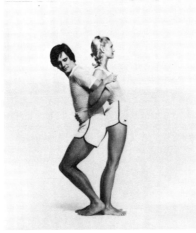

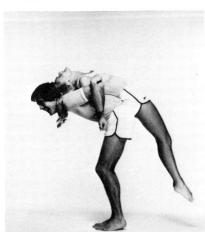

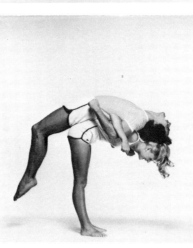

Pullovers This is terrific for tummy strength, your back and balance.

Stand back to back, holding hands at shoulder level.

The taller partner should fit his bottom *under* that of the smaller partner.

The bigger partner leans forward, bending his knees, until the other body hangs free and relaxed. Hold for a few seconds, then straighten up slowly.

Repeat with the smaller partner taking the strain; do it three times each.

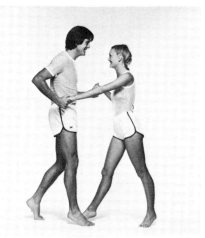

Scissors Good exercise for strengthening leg muscles (use it as an indoor form of jogging, when it's too wet to run outdoors).

Stand facing your partner, one foot slightly in front of the other, holding hands loosely with arms bent. Now 'scissor' both feet past each other sixteen times.

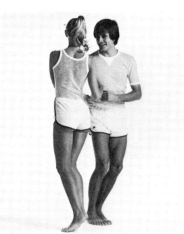

Twists This is great for waist and hips.

Stand facing your partner, feet together, holding hands lightly. Now twist your body from left to right (opposite directions) from the *waist down* only, keeping your chest facing forward. Count sixteen, then relax.

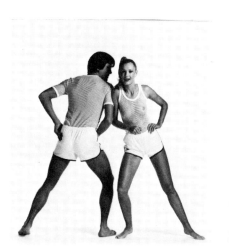

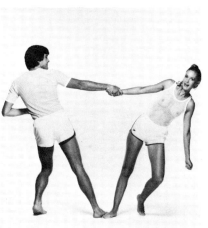

Push me, pull you This one develops strength in your arms, back, tummy, legs and feet.

Stand facing each other with the outsides of your right feet against each other, legs apart. Place your right upper arms and shoulders together, and push. Hold for a count of three, change sides and push again.

Now grasp each other's right wrists and *pull*. Hold for a count of three, change hands and repeat. Do four sets.

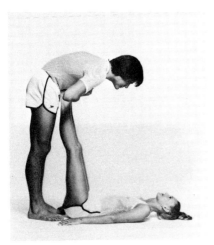
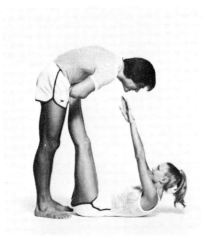

Shoulder sit-ups Excellent for your tummy and those underworked hamstring muscles.

Lie on the floor on your back, feet stretched up to your partner's waist. Get him to hold your ankles, and lean forward slightly to 'anchor' your legs.

Now, raise your head and shoulders off the floor and stretch your fingertips towards his shoulders. Hold for a count of six, then relax slowly. Repeat six times, then swap over and repeat a further six times.

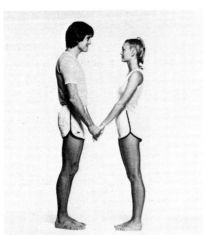
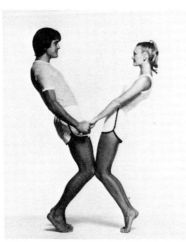

Knees-up Super for your feet, calves, quadriceps and tummy muscles.

Face each other, holding hands, elbows bent, feet and knees tightly together.

Contract buttock and tummy muscles, and rise up on your toes, tilting your pelvis forward and pressing your knees forward until they touch. Hold for a count of three (no wobbling) then, very slowly, lower your heels. Repeat ten times.

Legometrics

Many women have problems with wobbly thighs, thick calves and bulging ankles, mainly caused by lack of muscle use and fluid retention. Beautiful legs do need exercise, so walk as much as possible and do the six sensational exercises below every night. To beat the fluid problem, try lying down flat on the floor with your bottom against the wall and your legs at right-angles to your body, ankles resting on the wall, for about ten minutes every evening. Avoid tight shoes and don't sit around drinking tea all day!

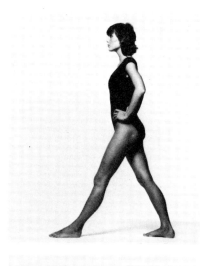 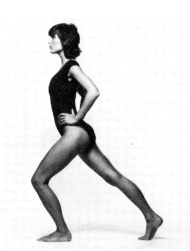

1 With hands on your hips, stand with right leg straight out in front, left leg straight out behind. Check that your weight is evenly distributed between your feet.

Now, bend your right leg, moving your weight on to it. Keep your back straight and lower your body as far as possible without leaning forward. Bend and straighten up twenty times, swap legs and repeat.

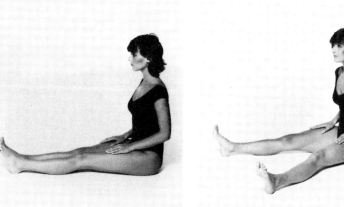 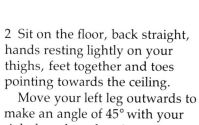

2 Sit on the floor, back straight, hands resting lightly on your thighs, feet together and toes pointing towards the ceiling.

Move your left leg outwards to make an angle of 45° with your right leg, then close it again. Repeat movement with right leg, then repeat double movement ten times.

3 Lie on your right side on the floor with your head resting on your right hand, left hand supporting your weight on the floor in front of you.

Raise your left leg about one inch off the floor and hold in this position.

Bend left leg in towards stomach, then straighten out rapidly. Do the last two movements twenty times, then change sides and repeat a further twenty times.

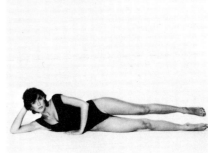

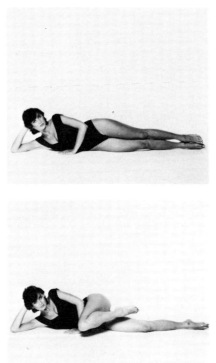

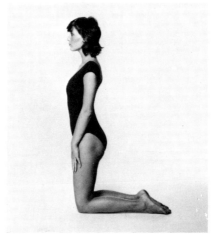

4 Kneel on the floor, knees slightly apart, hands resting on the front of your thighs.

Now lean back as far as you can without arching your back. Feel that pull on your thigh muscles? Repeat fifteen times.

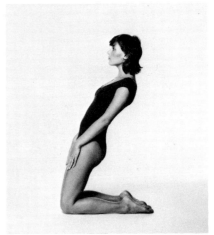

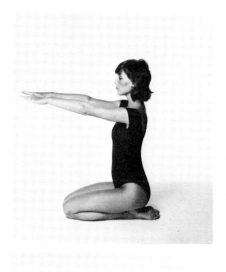

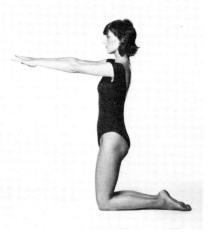

5 Sit back on your heels on the floor, keeping arms straight out in front.

Now rise up, straightening your body.

Lower your bottom to a sitting position to the left of your heels.

Rise up again.

This time lower your bottom to a sitting position to the right of your heels. Repeat complete movement ten times.

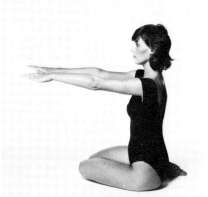

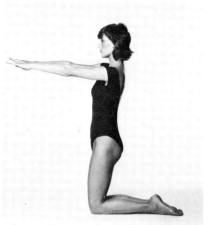

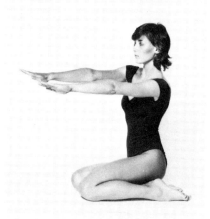

6 Lie on your back, hands by your sides, palms down for support.

Raise your knees to your chest.

Stretch your legs straight up.

Hold the position briefly, then let them fall apart as far as they will go, then close them together. Open and close six times, then bend your knees back to your chest, and lower your legs slowly. Repeat the whole movement five times.

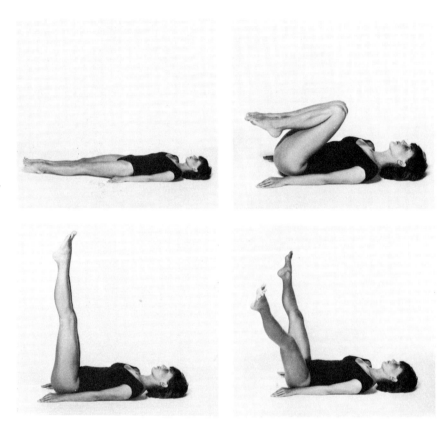

Jazz–dance exercises

You've got rhythm! Don't believe it? However clumsy you think you are, there's a whole new breed of dance and fitness experts who aim to prove that you can shimmy, shake, jive and boogie your way to a beautiful figure. Dance exercise classes are springing up all over the country – it's fun doing it to music! If you don't feel quite ready to expose your lack of timing to other people straight away, try the routines below in the privacy of your bedroom first.

The first two exercises consist of controlled movements to do to a fairly slow record (blues would be good); the others are faster and should be performed as a sequence to rapid music. Try reggae to start off with, then work up to heavy rock! Best of all, use these exercises as a basis for your own disco routine.

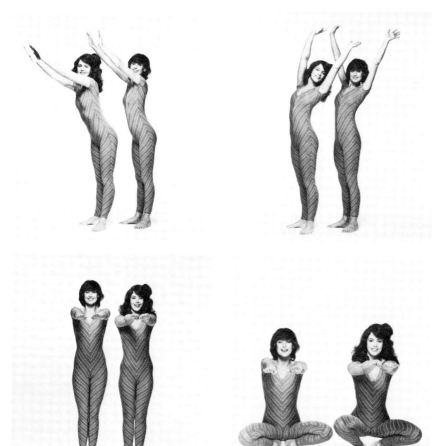

Warm-up Stand with feet slightly apart and turned out, arms and shoulders relaxed. Now raise your arms above your head, tuck your tum and bottom in and bend forward and back (keep those arms and shoulders relaxed). Do twenty to forty movements, speeding up as you go. Helps straighten that vulnerable lower back, and stretches your torso like crazy.

Knees-bend Stand on your toes, heels together, arms outstretched for balance. Now pushing your heels together, bend your knees open wide, and squeeze your buttock muscles together. Try and stay on your tip-toes, but lower heels if you must as you bend. Start with eight to ten movements, keeping your back absolutely straight.

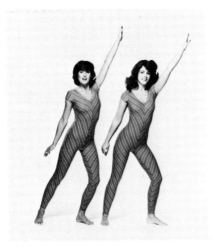 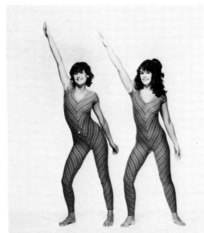

Stretch-up Legs apart, back straight, look up at the ceiling. Now reach up with your right arm, leaning into your right knee. Repeat with your left arm, left knee (it feels like climbing). Keep it up until you feel stretched, refreshed.

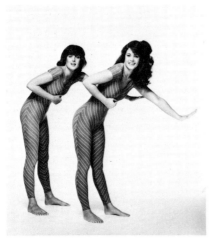 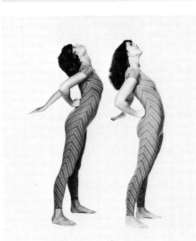

Rib-tickler Stand straight, feet apart. Stretch your left hand, palm down, in front of you. Hunch your shoulders, poke your right index finger into your chest, exhale, and 'curl' your ribs around your finger. Then push the thumb of the same hand into the middle of your back, inhale, opening ribs and flinging left hand behind you. Now try it with the other finger. Keep repeating the movement with alternate hands until you've worked up a good rhythm. Super for shoulders, ribs, posture.

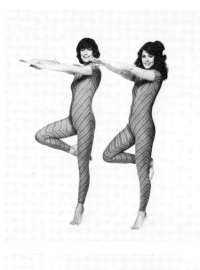

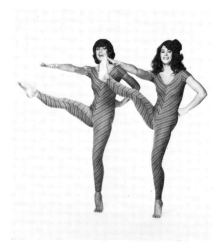

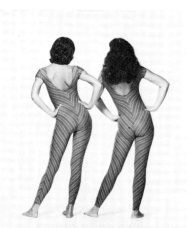

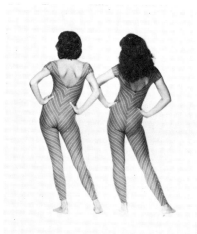

Just for kicks Stand with feet together, arms raised in front of your chest, elbows bent. Now draw your right knee up, right foot hooked behind your left leg, both knees bent. Kick straight out in front of you, straightening both legs and pushing your right hand forward, left elbow back. Now drop leg so both feet are together on the floor. Bend knees and start again, kicking up alternate legs in a 'chorus line' movement. It works wonders for your legs, and increases stamina and strength.

Hip roll Stand with your feet slightly apart, hands on your hips, elbows out. Roll your right hip to the right, return to centre, then roll your left hip to the left. Return to centre. Repeat this figure-of-eight movement for one minute, keeping your knees bent and working up a good rhythm. Remember to keep your tummy muscles tucked in and your bottom tight and high. It's great for your hips, thighs, tum, waistline.

The big three

What's your biggest problem area? I bet it's either your tummy, bosom or bottom. If they are wobbly, flabby or out of shape, your whole body feels less than perfect, even though you may be the correct weight for your height and body type. Luckily, all three respond well to intensive exercises (yes, even your bosom can look lots better with exercise; small bosoms have been known to *grow* when on the receiving end of a little attention!) which needn't be too time-consuming. Try one of the three exercise plans below for a week and just see the difference!

Flat tummy plan To encourage those flabby muscles to *work*, for a change, don't encase your tummy in tight jeans. Instead, make this the week you wear a skirt or dress that's just a bit revealing so you *have* to hold your tummy in. While you're sitting or standing, hold those muscles right in for a count of ten, then release slowly – do this every hour on the hour, all day long wherever you happen to be. Now, try these three exercises every day:

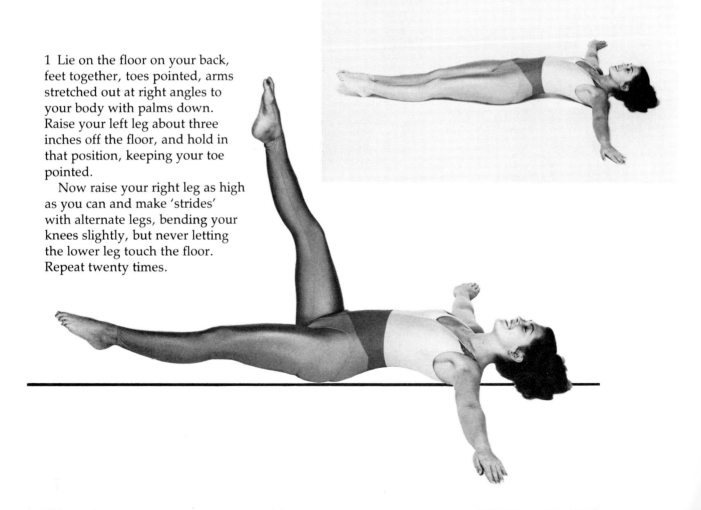

1 Lie on the floor on your back, feet together, toes pointed, arms stretched out at right angles to your body with palms down. Raise your left leg about three inches off the floor, and hold in that position, keeping your toe pointed.

Now raise your right leg as high as you can and make 'strides' with alternate legs, bending your knees slightly, but never letting the lower leg touch the floor. Repeat twenty times.

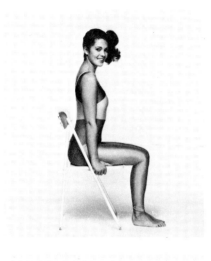
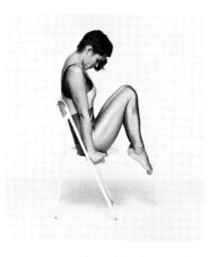

2 Sit on a chair, knees bent, feet together. Hold the seat of the chair with both hands. Now drop your chin on to your chest, lift your knees and point your toes (back straight). Hold for a count of two, then lower your toes to the ground and raise your head. Breathing is important in this one: breathe *out*, pulling your tummy right in as you lift your knees, breathe *in* as you lower them. Repeat ten times.

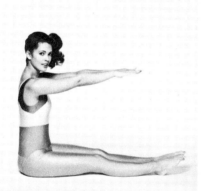
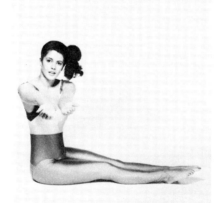

3 Sit on the floor, legs and arms straight in front, back straight, stomach muscles pulled in.

Fling your arms smoothly to the right side of your body, palms uppermost, twisting your trunk to the right as you move.

Now swing back to the forward position, and lean forward to touch your toes (or knees!) with both hands. Raise your trunk to the upright position, bringing your hands up to chest-level. Do five sets to the right, then five to the left, keep all movements smooth and flowing.

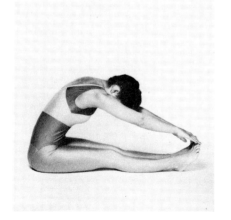

Beautiful bosom plan Bosom too small or too droopy? Exercise can help strengthen the pectoral muscles, which support the breasts and make your bosom look higher and bigger. Psychologists report that some women seem able to make their breasts increase in size with concentration, daily massage and loving care. It is certainly true that girls who pay more attention to their bosom shape than most women seem able to improve the size and look of their breasts over a few months. Being in love is one way to make your chest look splendid; the breast tissue actually expands by up to forty per cent during lovemaking, the pectorals contract, the nipples lengthen; the whole thing constitutes a super natural 'exercise' for your bust.

What if your bust is too big? If it's large and droopy, it can look very unattractive. If it's big and beautiful, then you're a very lucky lady. The best plan is to exercise to keep your pectorals toned up, wear a flattering bra and make sure your *posture* is immaculate. You should make a real effort to sit and stand with your shoulders well back and to walk correctly (especially if you have to carry heavy shopping). Do these exercises every day:

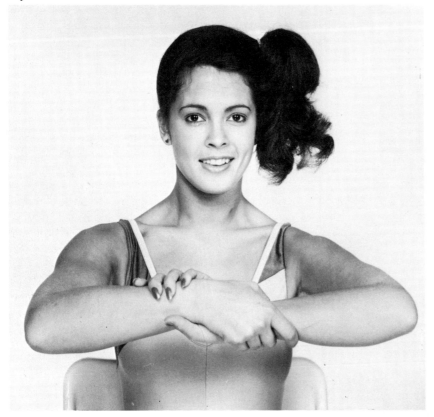

1 Sit or stand with your elbows raised, hands clasping your wrists in front of your chest. Now push sharply away from your wrists towards your elbows, moving the flesh itself *not* the position of your hands. If you're doing it correctly you should feel your pectorals twitching and see your breasts rise. Repeat fifty times (in the bath is a good place).

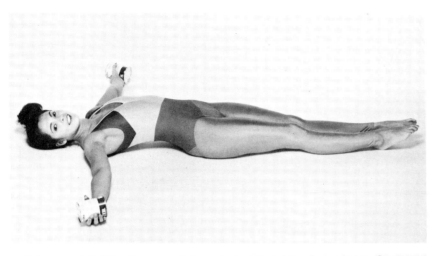

2 Lie on your back on the floor, feet together, arms stretched out at right angles to your body with a weight such as a baked bean tin (full!) in each hand.

Fling your arms across your chest then out to each side in a rapid scissor movement. Repeat fifty times.

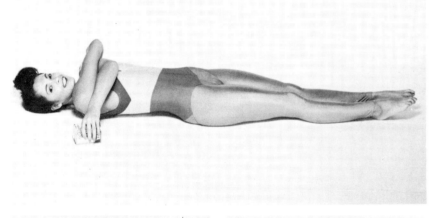

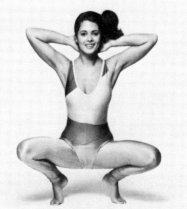

3 Stand with your feet wide apart, hands on the back of your neck. Now squat, keeping your back straight, elbows well out and your weight on your heels. Straighten up, breathing in, and push your hands against the back of your neck, elbows out. Repeat five times.

Trim bottom plan A bulging bottom can be a big problem, especially if it's flabby or low-slung! Unfortunately, nature is very unkind; women are programmed to store fat around the bottom and hips as protection for their childbearing regions. That's why any surplus weight is so often directed by the body's fat mobilizing mechanism towards its favourite target area – your rear. What can you do about it? Try using your buttock muscles more often. It's tricky to do this, since these muscles are best exercised by contraction and backward leg movements. If you sit in an office all day on a squashy chair, and in an equally squashy chair all evening, they simply don't have to contract at all. Just for one week, try *making* your muscles contract; pulling them in tightly, count six then release. Repeat this twenty times every hour, and do the exercises below every day. You should also increase the amount of walking you do, taking long determined strides to maximize the muscle movement. Walk *backwards* (upstairs!) too, if you have time.

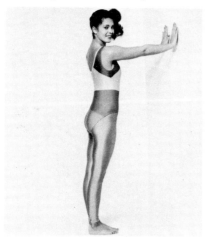

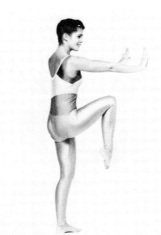

1 Stand at arms' distance from a wall, with feet together, palms flat against the wall and arms straight.

Raise one knee to your chest.

Now stretch the leg downwards and swing it backwards as high as you can, keeping your trunk straight (you mustn't lean forward). Do it five times with one leg, then five with the other.

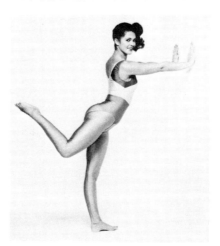

2 Kneel on all fours, hands and knees slightly apart, head up.

Bring one knee up to touch your nose (or as near as possible).

Now straighten that leg, swinging it up and back and as high as possible. Do it five times with one leg, then five with the other.

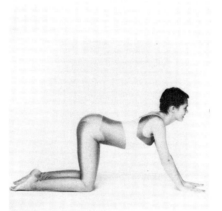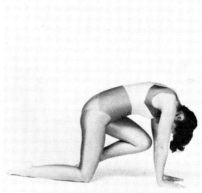

3 Lie on the floor on your tummy, feet together, arms by your sides, toes pointed.

Now raise one leg (keep it straight) as high as you can, cross it over your other leg, and lower to touch the floor. Using alternate legs repeat the whole movement as many times as you can, building up to fifty.

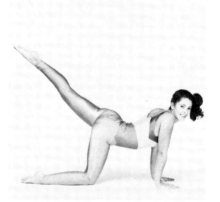

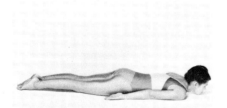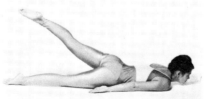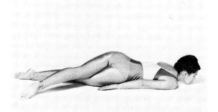

Slimming Addresses

Health farms and clubs

Champneys
Tring
Hertfordshire
Berkhamsted 73155/6

Medically-supervised dieting and exercising programme, especially suitable for men. Physiotherapy, yoga, lectures, relaxation classes, indoor and outdoor sports, luxury accommodation.

Chevin Hall
Otley
West Yorkshire
Otley 462526

Moderately priced with balanced diets, beauty treatments. Their speciality is a five-day course.

Forest Mere
Liphook
Hampshire
Liphook 722051

Underwater massage, physiotherapy, osteopathy, faradic and galvanic slimming treatments, swimming pools, beauty treatments including cathiodermie.

Grayshott Hall
Grayshott
Hindhead
Surrey
Hindhead 4331

Faradic and galvanic slimming treatments, underwater massage, games room, gym, solarium, osteopathy, yoga, skin conditioning treatments including cathiodermie, bio-peel and vapozone.

Henlow Grange
Henlow
Bedfordshire
Hitchin 811111

Exercise classes, paraffin wax treatments, solarium, Swedish massage, hydrotherapy, sports facilities, beauty and hairdressing.

Holmes Place Health Club
188 Fulham Road
London SW10
01–352 9452

Gym, studio, steam room, sauna, whirlpools. Dance, yoga, self-defence. Restaurant and shop. Membership only.

Inglewood Health Hydro
Kintbury
Berkshire
Hungerford 2022

Luxury stately home with facilities for osteopathy, electrotherapy, physiotherapy, massage, sauna, steam baths, hydrotherapy; medically supervised.

Kilkea Castle
Castledermont
County Kildare
Ireland
Carlow 45156

Luxury castle with separate sections for men and women. Sauna, gymnasium, plunge pools; full range of beauty treatments and diets.

Ragdale Hall
Ragdale
Melton Mowbray
Leicestershire
Melton Mowbray 75831

Faradic, galvanic and mud slimming treatments, gym, underwater massage, aromatherapy, beauty treatments, cathiodermie and bio-peel. Moderately priced with excellent diets.

The Sanctuary
Floral Street
London WC2
01–836 6544

Club for women only with day membership including use of gym, swimming pool, sauna, solarium. Dance classes and beauty treatments also available.

Shenley Lodge
Ridge Hill
Radlett
Hertfordshire
Potters Bar 42424/5

Moderately priced with diets, beauty treatments, exercises to music, hairdressing. They specialize in long weekend sessions.

Shrublands Hall Health Clinic
Coddenham
Ipswich
Suffolk
Ipswich 830404

Medium price-range with full health and beauty facilities, authoritative dietary advice.

Stobo Castle
Peeblesshire
Scotland
Peebles 6249

Luxury castle just outside Edinburgh catering for twenty-six guests a week. Resident dietician, full range of beauty treatments and hairdressing; yoga, reflexology, aromatherapy, spot reduction and massage.

Tyringham Naturopathic Clinic
Newport Pagnell
Buckinghamshire
Newport Pagnell 610450

Stringent vegetarian diet,
therapeutic hydrotherapy,
acupuncture, osteopathy, yoga,
sauna, sports facilities.

Westside Health Centre
201–7 Kensington High Street
London W8
01–937 5386

Club with day membership
including use of sauna, gym,
specialized dietary advice,
movement classes, special rates
for squash and swimming pool.

Exercise and dance studios

Corinthian Health Studio
41 Smallbrook
Queensway
Birmingham
021–643 8712

Gym, sauna, solarium and beauty
salon.

Corinthian Health Studio
215a Old Christchurch Road
Bournemouth
Hampshire
Bournemouth 28755

Gym, sauna, solarium and beauty
salon.

Dick Hubbard Fitness Centre
Packhorse Walk
Huddersfield
Yorkshire
Huddersfield 49025

Gym, sauna, solarium, exercise
classes.

Dance Centre
11–12 Floral Street
London WC2
01–836 6544

All types of dance class.

Gym 'n' Tonic
4 Welbeck Street
London W1
01–580 4556

Gym, sauna, whirlpool, health
bar; half-hour work-out classes at
lunchtime and after work hours.

London School of Contemporary
   Dance
16 Flaxman Terrace
London WC1
01–387 0161

Classes in contemporary dance
and exercise.

Lotte Berk
29 Manchester Street
London W1
01–935 8905

Classes of very strenuous ballet
movements, bar and floor work.

N. W. Health
26 Barrow Street
St Helens
Lancashire
St Helens 32535

Gym, fitness training, sunbeds,
sauna.

N. W. Health
Library Street
Wigan
Lancashire
Wigan 31439

Gym, fitness training, sunbeds,
sauna.

Keep Fit Association
70 Brompton Road
London SW3
01–584 3271

Contact this address for the club
in your area.

Outline Figure & Fitness Club
21/31 Old Street
Manchester
061–832 2555

Gym, sauna, solarium and beauty
salon.

Outline Figure & Fitness Club
Mersey Square
Stockport
Greater Manchester
061–477 0160

Gym, sauna, solarium, beauty
salon, exercise and slimming
programme.

Dick Hubbard Outline Figure &
   Fitness Club
Union Street
Oldham
Lancashire
061–652 7418

Gym, sauna, solarium, exercise
classes. Personal programme
worked out by computer.

Pineapple Dance Centre
7 Langley Street
London WC2
01–836 4004

Every type of dance and exercise class from classic to disco; for beginners and professionals.

YMCA
112 Gt Russell Street
London WC1
01–637 8131

Exercise classes, classical ballet, mime and disco. Also swimming pool, sports facilities, sauna and solarium.

Slimming clubs

Silhouette Slimming Club
103 Harlestone Road
Northampton
Northampton 53921

Slenderquest
117 High Street
Barnet
01–441 4688

Slimming Magazine Clubs
4 Clareville Grove
London SW7
01–370 4411

The Slimnastics Association
14 East Sheen Avenue
London SW14
01–876 1838

Society of Serious Slimmers
37 Cadogan Street
London SW3
01–589 3557

Weight-Watchers
635–7 Ajax Avenue
Slough
Berkshire
Slough 70711

London Women's Therapy Centre
  (for compulsive eaters)
6 Manor Gardens
London N7
01–263 6200

Beauty salons specializing in slimming treatments

Harrods
Knightsbridge
London SW1
01–730 1234

Body massage, sauna and cellulite treatments.

Hawkins Clinic 42 Beauchamp Place London SW3 *01–589 1853*	Galvanic and faradic slimming treatments, aromatherapy, body massage, cellulite treatments.
Marguerite Maury Suite 101 Park Lane Hotel London W1 *01–499 6321*	Aromatherapy massage and slimming advice.
Marietta Kavanagh 4a William Street London SW1 *01–235 4106*	Cellulite treatments, massage, facials, dietary advice.
Micheline Arcier 4 Albert Gate Court 124 Knightsbridge London SW1 *01–589 3225*	Aromatherapy body massage, slimming advice. For women only.
Morlé Slimming and Beauty Centre 176 Kensington High Street London W8 *01–937 9501*	Cellulite and stretch mark treatments, aromatherapy, gym, sauna.
Town and Country Health and Beauty Salon	Full slimming and beauty course arranged according to your needs.

2 Yeoman's Row
London SW3
01–584 7702

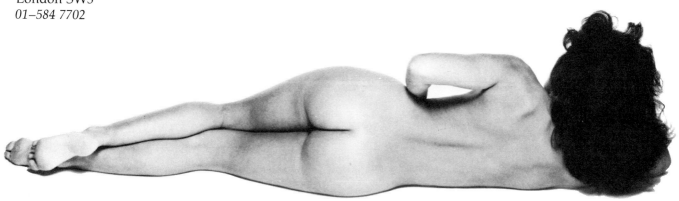

Index